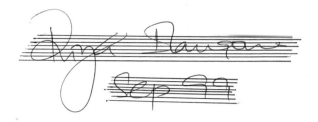

An Atlas of
EPILEPSY

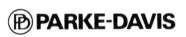

This copy of 'An Atlas of Epilepsy'
is presented to the department

of ....

as a service to Medicine by

℗ PARKE-DAVIS

OVER 50 YEARS' EXPERIENCE IN THE
MANAGEMENT OF EPILEPSY

THE ENCYCLOPEDIA OF VISUAL MEDICINE SERIES

An Atlas of
EPILEPSY

D.F. Smith, MD, MRCP, R.E. Appleton, MA(Oxon), FRCP,
J.M. MacKenzie, MBChB(Ed), FRCPath, and D.W. Chadwick, DM, FRCP

Walton Centre for Neurology and Neurosurgery, Liverpool;
Roald Dahl EEG Unit, Alder Hey Children's Hospital, Liverpool;
Department of Pathology, Medical School, Foresterhill, Aberdeen Royal Hospital Trust, Aberdeen;
and University Department of Neurosciences, University of Liverpool, Liverpool; UK

Foreword by

Richard H. Mattson, MD

Department of Neurology, Yale University School of Medicine,
New Haven, Connecticut, USA

The Parthenon Publishing Group
International Publishers in Medicine, Science & Technology

NEW YORK   LONDON

Library of Congress Cataloging-in-Publication Data
An atlas of epilepsy / D.F. Smith. . . . [et al..].
       p.   cm — (The Encyclopedia of visual medicine series)
    Includes bibliographical references and index.
    ISBN 1-85070-488-0
    1. Epilepsy--Atlases. I. Smith, D.F. (David F.). 1960–
II. Series.
    [DNLM: 1. Epilepsy--atlases. WL 17 A8833 1997]
RC372,A85 1997--
616.8'53'00222--dc21
DNLM/DLC
for Library of Congress   97–987
                                                        CIP

British Library Cataloguing-in-Publication Data
An atlas of epilepsy. – (The encyclopedia of visual medicine
     series)
     1. Epilepsy – Atlases
     I. Smith, D.F.
     616.8'53

ISBN 1-85070-488-0

Published in the USA by
The Parthenon Publishing Group Inc.
One Blue Hill Plaza
PO Box 1564, Pearl River
New York 10965, USA

Published in the UK and Europe by
The Parthenon Publishing Group Limited
Casterton Hall, Carnforth
Lancs. LA6 2LA, UK

Copyright © 1998 Parthenon Publishing Group

First published 1998

Printed and bound in Spain by T.G. Hostench, S.A.

Contents

Foreword

As a worldwide medical problem affecting approximately 1% of the population, epilepsy has a prevalence comparable to that of insulin-dependent diabetes mellitus. Emerging from centuries of misunderstanding, epilepsy has benefitted, especially in recent decades, from a dramatic increase in knowledge of the etiologies, pathophysiology, clinical types, diagnostic methods and treatment.

Although excellent textbooks and monographs have been published elucidating these various aspects of epilepsy, few provide extensive visual illustrations. *An Atlas of Epilepsy* comprises a text accompanied by illustrations of the pathology as well as selected electroencephalographic recordings and diagnostic images. Complementary graphs and diagrams, specially prepared for inclusion in this book, render helpful depictions of the etiologies, prognosis and treatment of epilepsy. The superb quality of the figures brings out the essential elements with great clarity.

The beautiful and well-selected illustrations in this atlas make this volume not only informative, but also enjoyable to use. Although the illustrations are of primary importance, the written text offers a salient counterpart. The first six chapters briefly, but comprehensively, present information regarding the fundamentals of epilepsy. Selected references guide the reader to additional resources for greater detail.

An Atlas of Epilepsy will be a valued addition to medical libraries and to those who have an interest in epilepsy.

Richard H. Mattson, MD
New Haven

Preface

Hughlings Jackson defined epilepsy as "the expression of occasional, sudden, excessive, rapid local discharges in the gray matter"; he could not have foreseen the evolution and transfiguration of what is primarily a functional disorder into the striking and vivid series of visual images which it now represents.

Epilepsy is now regarded as much more than a functional disorder of the central nervous system; it is in fact a collection of conditions with different pathophysiologies, multiple manifestations and diverse etiologies.

There is now a considerable amount of information regarding the epidemiology, natural history and prognosis of the epilepsies, much of which can be illustrated simply, but effectively, in graphic form. The increasing technological sophistication and understanding of the basic mechanisms and causes of epileptic seizures emphasize the importance of the visual aspects of epilepsy.

The electroencephalogram (EEG), which allows the pictorial display of abnormal cerebral activity, is central to the classification of the epilepsies and epilepsy syndromes. Computed tomography and magnetic resonance imaging have revealed not only the obvious, but also the many subtle, structural abnormalities in the brain responsible for seizures, as well as their susceptibility to surgical treatment. Advances in positron emission tomography and single-photon emission tomography are increasingly allowing the production of 'functional' images of the brain that are particularly relevant to epileptogenesis.

The treatment of epilepsy has, since the time of Hughlings Jackson, improved dramatically with the advent of more effective and less toxic antiepileptic drugs, and the development of specialist multidisciplinary services. More specifically, surgical ablation of epileptic foci has vividly demonstrated the marked neuropathological heterogeneity of the epilepsies.

An Atlas of Epilepsy provides the first pictorial representation of this most common and chronic disorder of the central nervous system, and also complements the already published textbooks on epilepsy by adding a new, hitherto unexplored, perspective on this group of conditions. This book and its approach to epilepsy should be of interest and value to all those who are involved with the subject.

David F. Smith
Richard E. Appleton
James M. MacKenzie
David W. Chadwick
Liverpool and Aberdeen

Acknowledgements

The authors would like to thank the following individuals for their invaluable help and contributions to this project:

Mrs Linda Finnegan, Mrs Margaret Beirne, and Mrs Barbara Acomb, The Roald Dahl EEG Unit, Royal Liverpool Children's Hospital, Alder Hey, Liverpool; Professor Helen Carty, Consultant Pediatric Radiologist, Royal Liverpool Children's Hospital, Alder Hey, Liverpool; Professor John Stephenson, Consultant Pediatric Neurologist, Royal Hospital for Sick Children, Glasgow; Dr C.P. Panayiotopoulos, Consultant in Clinical Neurophysiology, St. Thomas' Hospital, London; Drs N.R. Clitheroe, T.E. Nixon and E.T. Smith, Neuroradiologists, Walton Centre for Neurology and Neurosurgery, Liverpool; Dr R. Duncan, Consultant Neurologist, Southern General Hospital, Glasgow; Mr T. Lesser, Consultant ENT Surgeon, Aintree Hospital NHS Trust, Liverpool; and Dr Helen Cross, Institute of Child Health and Great Ormond Street Hospital for Children NHS Trust, London.

Section 1 A Review of Epilepsy

1 Definitions and basic mechanisms

Definitions

Seizures and epilepsy are clinical phenomena resulting from hyperexcitability of the neurons of the cerebral hemispheres. They may be defined in both physiological and clinical terms:

Physiologically, epilepsy is the name for occasional sudden, excessive, rapid and local discharges of gray matter. Up-to-date evidence indicates that increased and hypersynchronous neuronal discharges are the essential features involved in the generation of seizures.

Clinically, an epileptic seizure is an intermittent stereotypical, usually unprovoked, disturbance of consciousness, behavior, emotion, motor function or sensation that is the result of cortical neuronal discharge. Epilepsy is a condition in which seizures recur, usually spontaneously.

Basic mechanisms of epilepsy

There are fundamental physiological differences between focal and generalized epileptogenesis, which probably explain their wide range of clinical manifestations and varied responses to different antiepileptic agents.

Focal epileptogenesis

The cellular correlate of the interictal spike wave is a paroxysmal depolarization shift (PDS) of the resting membrane potential, which triggers a brief rapid burst of action potentials terminated by a sustained after-hyperpolarization (Figure 1). The PDS may be the result either of an imbalance between excitatory (glutamate and aspartate) and inhibitory (gamma-aminobutyric acid; GABA) neurotransmitters or of abnormalities of voltage-controlled membrane ion channels. Increased sodium and calcium conductance, and reduced potassium conductance favor depolarization and burst firing.

Asynchronous burst-firing occurs spontaneously in some hippocampal and cortical neurons. Synchronization of neuronal burst behavior and propagation of epileptic discharges require both impaired inhibition and intact excitatory synaptic connections. The initiation of focal epileptogenesis is probably due to an imbalance between endogenous neuromodulators, with acetylcholine favoring depolarization and dopamine enhancing neuronal membrane stability.

Knowledge of the structure of neurotransmitter receptors provides a means of understanding the modes of action of conventional antiepileptic drugs

Table 1.1 Pharmacological enhancement of GABA-mediated inhibition

Mechanism	Compound
True GABA agonist	
GABA$_A$ receptor	muscimol
GABA$_B$ receptor	baclofen
GABA prodrug	progabide
Stimulation of GABA synthesis	milacemide
Allosteric enhancement of GABA efficacy	benzodiazepines anticonvulsant beta-carbolines
Direct action on chloride ionophore	phenobarbitone
Inhibition of GABA re-uptake	nipecotic acid
Inhibition of GABA transaminase	vigabatrin

and serves as a basis for the rational development of new antiepileptic agents.

GABA$_A$ receptor and chloride ion channel

GABA is the major inhibitory neurotransmitter in the central nervous system. There is compelling evidence that loss of postsynaptic GABA-mediated inhibition is crucial to the gewnesis of focal seizures.

Activation of the GABA$_A$ receptor (Figure 2) opens the chloride channel on the GABA/benzodiazepine complex, allowing chloride influx, hyperpolarization of the postsynaptic neuron and inhibition of firing.

Several antiepileptic drugs (and experimental compounds) exert their antiepileptic effects via mechanisms which enhance GABA-mediated inhibition (Table 1.1). Vigabatrin, a suicidal inhibitor of GABA transaminase, was the first antiepileptic drug to be developed with a specific mode of action.

NMDA receptor and calcium channel

Glutamate is the predominant excitatory neurotransmitter in the nervous system. Four postsynaptic receptor subtypes can be identified, according to preferential binding of endogenous ligands.

The N-methyl-D-aspartate (NMDA) receptor (Figure 3) is most likely to have a role in epilepsy. Stimulation of this receptor produces an intracellular cationic flux, particularly calcium, with rapid depolarization and sustained repetitive firing. NMDA antagonists are potent anticonvulsants in animal models, but their clinical evaluation has been limited by neurotoxicity.

However, excitatory neurotransmission can be manipulated in other ways (Table 1.2). The novel antiepileptic drug lamotrigine acts via inhibition of the release of glutamate presynaptically.

Voltage-sensitive sodium channels

A number of conventional (phenytoin and carbamazepine) and novel antiepileptic drugs (lamotrigine) act by voltage-dependent modulation of sodium channels. This involves a shift in steady-state inactivation to hyperpolarized membrane voltages. This shift has been experimentally demonstrated for both phenytoin and lamotrigine. Consequently, drug-bound inactivated sodium channels cannot easily return to the resting state, thereby preventing conduction of sodium, depolarization and sustained repetitive firing.

Table 1.2 Pharmacological approaches to decrease glutamatergic neurotransmission

Mechanism	Compound
Decreased glutamate synthesis (glutaminase inhibitors)	aserazine
Decreased presynaptic glutamate release	adenosine analog lamotrigine
Postsynaptic receptor antagonists	
non-selective	kynurenic acid
selective NMDA antagonists	
competitive	CPP
non-competitive	MK801
	remacemide
kainate / quisqualate antagonists	
metabotropic receptor antagonists	
Enhanced glutamate uptake	
Long-term downregulation of the excitatory amino acid (EAA) system	

CPP, 3-[(*)-2-carboxy-piperazin-4-YL]propyl-1-phosphonate

Generalized epileptogenesis

The generalized spike-and-wave (GSW) seizure is produced by an abnormal thalamocortical interaction which oscillates between enhanced excitation with firing (spike wave) and enhanced inhibition with hyperpolarization (slow wave). In humans, the primary abnormality is cortical hyperexcitability, which may be due to a genetically determined metabolic defect or a minor morphological abnormality such as microdysgenesis.

There is strong evidence that generalized epileptogenesis is mediated via calcium T channels, which are found in high density in thalamic neurons and activated by relatively low-voltage thresholds after sustained depolarization. The resultant low-threshold calcium current (LTCC) generates a low-threshold calcium spike (LTCS), which underlies the slow thalamic rhythms seen in 3-cps GSW or absence seizures. The selective blockade of calcium T channels is the likely mechanism of action of antiabsence drugs such as ethosuximide.

2 Epidemiology

Epilepsy is the most common of the neurological disorders. The most complete epidemiological study, from Rochester, Minnesota, reports an age- and gender-adjusted annual incidence of 49 per 100 000 population, with peaks both in the first year of life and in senescence, and a lifetime cumulative incidence of 3% by age 80 years (Figure 4).

The most recent data define a prevalence of 6.8/1000 population, which suggests that approximately 400 000 subjects in the UK and 2 000 000 in the USA have active epilepsy. The large and ever-increasing gap between point prevalence and lifetime cumulative incidence is a reflection, in many cases, of the self-limiting nature of the condition.

The age-adjusted annual death rate for epilepsy varies widely among countries (0.4–4/100 000), perhaps due to differences in prevalence rates and/or different methods of recording on death certificates. The factors associated with a higher mortality include male gender, age (< 1 year, > 50 years), marital status (single) and epilepsy symptomatic of diffuse or focal cerebral disease.

The standardized mortality ratio for epilepsy is high (Table 2.1). In approximately 25% of cases, death may be related to seizures (status epilepticus, accidental injury and sudden unexplained death). Suicide and cerebral tumors are over-represented as causes of death in patients with epilepsy.

Table 2.1 Standardized mortality ratios for patients with epilepsy in the Rochester study (1935–1974) by etiology of the epilepsy and follow-up period

Years of follow-up	Total	Idiopathic	Neurodeficit since birth	Potentially acquired secondary epilepsy
0–1	3.8	2.5	20.0	4.3
2–4	2.4	1.7	33.3	2.0
5–9	2.0	2.4	2.0	1.6
10–19	1.4	1.1	6.7	1.1
20–29	2.4	2.0	10.0	3.3
Total	2.3	1.8	11.0	2.2

With permission, from Hauser WA, Annegers JF, Elveback LR. Mortality in patients with epilepsy. *Epilepsia* 1980;**21**:399–412

3 Diagnosis

The diagnosis of epilepsy is a three-step process, consisting of the differential diagnosis, classification of seizures and epilepsy, and definition of the cause.

Differential diagnosis

Differentiation of seizures from other paroxysmal disorders with or without loss of consciousness can usually be achieved on clinical grounds alone, but may be difficult in some cases, particularly in young children.

The patient's history should include a detailed account of the symptoms before, during (if consciousness retained) and after the event(s) as well as the circumstances surrounding the attacks and, in particular, a clear eye-witness description. If diagnostic doubt remains, a policy of 'wait-and-see' should be adopted, as the diagnosis will usually be revealed by further events. Patients (or their parents if appropriate) should be asked to make a record, in written detail, of all further episodes and to present this information at subsequent reviews.

The use of a videocamera may be extremely useful in diagnosing epileptic *vs* non-epileptic paroxysmal events and may compensate for inadequate or inaccurate histories from eye-witnesses. In addition, on occasions, recording the symptomatic events with continuous ambulatory electroencephalography (EEG) monitoring will allow the differentiation of epileptic from non-epileptic attacks.

Neonatal seizures may be both over- and under-diagnosed. Generalized tonic-clonic seizures do not occur in neonates, in whom most seizures are localized (focal), fragmentary clonic, tonic or myoclonic. Many seizures are subtle and consist only of abnormal movement patterns such as mouthing / chewing, bicycling or boxing, or apnea and, thus, may easily go unrecognized.

Not all abnormal movements are seizures. The resultant difficulty in seizure recognition is greatest in premature infants. EEG reordings (specifically with simultaneous videorecording of clinical events) may resolve some of the difficulty, but there still remains the problem of 'electroclinical dissociation' in that electroencephalographically recognized seizures have an uncertain and inconstant relationship with clinical seizures.

Finally, a diagnosis of epilepsy in a child should be confirmed by a hospital clinician – a pediatrician, pediatric neurologist or adult neurologist – before investigations are performed or treatment initiated. The risk of a child with epilepsy coming to harm from a delay in diagnosis is minimal compared with the considerable potential and genuine harm that may arise from a false-positive diagnosis.

Table 3.1 Differential diagnosis of epilepsy in children

Episodes with altered consciousness	Episodes without altered consciousness
Delirium (with any febrile illness)	tics, rhythmic motor habits or mannerisms
Syncope (simple faint)	shuddering spells
Cyanotic ('blue') breath-holding attacks	rigors (with any febrile illness)
Pallid syncopal attacks (reflex anoxic seizures)	jitteriness (newborn period)
Night terrors	hypnagogic jerks (sleep myoclonus)
Migraine (the aura, or confusional and basilar	benign myoclonus of infancy
artery variants)	benign sleep myoclonus (neonatal and infantile)
Narcolepsy	benign familial paroxysmal kinesogenic choreoathetosis
Cardiac dysrhythmias	benign paroxysmal vertigo
prolonged QT syndrome	gastroesophageal reflux (Sandifer's syndrome)
Wolff–Parkinson–White syndrome	cardiac dysrhythmias
supraventricular tachycardias)	non-epileptic ('pseudo') seizures
Munchausen's syndrome by proxy (active)	Munchausen's syndrome by proxy (passive)

The differential diagnoses of epilepsy in children and in adults are summarized in Tables 3.1 and 3.2, respectively.

In children, simple faints (with or without brief hypoxic clonic seizures), migraine, night terrors, sleep myoclonus, cardiac dysrhythmias and tics/motor habits are commonly diagnosed as epilepsy (Table 3.1). Although no single feature differentiates these conditions from epilepsy, a careful account of the circumstances of the events should permit an accurate clinical diagnosis.

Pseudoseizures

The two most common phenomena causing misdiagnoses in adults are syncope and pseudoseizures or non-epileptic attacks (Tables 3.3 and 3.4).

Patients experiencing pseudoseizures or non-epileptic attacks constitute approximately 20% of the referrals to a specialist epilepsy clinic. Historical features which should alert the physician to this

Table 3.2 Differential diagnosis of epilepsy in adults

Syncope
Reflex syncope
    postural
    'psychogenic'
    micturition syncope
    Valsava
Cardiac syncope
    dysrhythmias (heart block, tachycardias, etc.)
    valvular disease (especially aortic stenosis)
    cardiomyopathies
    shunts
Perfusion failure
    hypovolemia
    syndrome of autonomic failure

Psychogenic attacks
Pseudoseizures
Panic attacks
Hyperventilation

Transient ischemic attacks

Migraine

Narcolepsy

Hypoglycemia

Table 3.3 Differences between syncope and seizures

Feature	Syncope	Seizure
Posture	upright	any posture
Pallor and sweating	invariable	uncommon
Onset	gradual	sudden / aura
Injury	rare	not uncommon
Convulsive jerks*	rare	common
Incontinence	rare	common
Unconsciousness†	seconds	minutes
Recovery	rapid	often slow
Postictal confusion	rare	common
Frequency	infrequent	may be frequent
Precipitating factors	crowded places, lack of food, unpleasant circumstances	rare

*Recent evidence indicates that brief myoclonic jerks occur in 80% of patients with syncope. Unlike an epileptic convulsion, however, recovery is rapid;

†Occasionally, syncope may result in a more prolonged period of cerebral hypoxia, which may cause an anoxic tonic-clonic seizure with a longer duration of unconsciousness and a slower rate of recovery

Table 3.4 Differences between epileptic seizures and pseudoseizures

Feature	Epileptic seizure	Pseudoseizure
Onset	sudden	may be gradual
Retained consciousness in prolonged seizure	very rare	common
Pelvic thrusting	rare	common
Flailing, thrashing, asynchronous limb movements	rare	common
Rolling movements	rare	common
Movements 'waxing and waning'	rare	common
Cyanosis	common	unusual
Tongue biting and other injury	common	less common
Stereotypical attacks	usual	uncommon
Duration	seconds or minutes	often many minutes
Gaze aversion	rare	common
Resistance to passive limb movement or eye-opening	unusual	common
Prevention of hand falling on face	unusual	common
Induced by suggestion	rarely	often
Postictal drowsiness or confusion	usual	often absent
Ictal EEG abnormality	almost always	almost never
Postictal EEG abnormality (after seizure with impairment of consciousness)	usually	rarely

Table 3.5 Factors associated with pseudoseizures / non-epileptic attacks

Attacks
Adult onset
Variable
Bizarre eye-witness descriptions
Circumstantial (provoked by stress)
Dramatic events
Recurrent hospitalization
No response or worse on antiepileptic drugs

Patient / past medical history
Female gender
Paramedical occupation
Traumatic childhood
Major life stressors (divorce, bereavement)
Past history of unexplained physical symptoms
Past psychiatric history, especially of self-abuse

Examination / investigation
Normal neurological examination
Evidence of illness behavior
EEG normal or non-specifically abnormal
CT scan normal

Table 3.6 Classification of seizures

Partial seizures (beginning locally)
Simple (consciousness unimpaired)
   with motor symptoms
   with somatosensory or special sensory symptoms
   with autonomic symptoms
   with psychic symptoms

Complex (consciousness impaired)
   beginning as simple partial seizures, but progressing
     to complex seizures
   with impaired consciousness at onset
      impairment of consciousness only
      with automatism

Partial but becoming secondarily generalized

Generalized seizures
Absence
   typical (petit mal)
   atypical
Myoclonic
Clonic
Tonic
Tonic-clonic
Atonic

From Commission on Classification and Terminology of the International League Against Epilepsy. Proposal for revised clinical and electroencephalographic classification of epilepsy seizures. *Epilepsia* 1981;**22**:489–501

diagnostic possibility are listed in Table 3.5. These patients may require admission to hospital for observation and ambulatory monitoring after stopping therapy and, when diagnosis is confirmed, referral for neuropsychological counselling;. An explanation is often evident in the family dynamics. If inappropriate antiepileptic drug therapy has not already been initiated, the patient management is simpler and the potentially disastrous psychosocial consequences may be avoided.

Classification of seizures and epilepsy

Epilepsy may be classified according to a number of different criteria, including severity, seizure type, etiology, anatomical localization, age at onset or EEG findings. Most of the classifications used in the past were based on one or more of these criteria and were entirely arbitrary, reflecting the limited understanding of the pathophysiology of epilepsy. In addition, these classifications have been virtually unusable in clinical practice.

At present, the most generally accepted classification of seizures (Table 3.6) classifies them according to whether their onset is focal (partial) or generalized. Partial seizures are further subdivided according to whether consciousness is retained throughout the seizure (simple partial) or impaired at some point (complex partial). Partial seizures are characterized by a warning, which has some localizing value, but any partial seizure can be secondarily generalized. In contrast, primarily generalized seizures occur with no warning.

Epilepsy syndromes

The concept of epileptic syndromes was first considered in 1985. In 1989, the International League Against Epilepsy (ILAE) revised the classification of epilepsy by incorporating epileptic syndromes in an attempt to simplify classification (Table 3.7).

A syndrome is a cluster of signs and symptoms that non-fortuitously occur together. An epileptic syndrome is characterized by both clinical and EEG findings:

Clinical findings
Seizure type(s)
Age at onset
Neurological findings
Family history;
EEG
Interictal
Ictal.

Delineation of the epileptic syndromes permits a greater precision of diagnosis and, more important, of prognosis than does the simple classification of seizure types. The same type of seizure can occur in different syndromes, but different types of seizure can also belong to the same syndrome.

The concept of epileptic syndromes is fundamentally pragmatic and helps in selecting the appropriate investigations, deciding on the optimal antiepileptic treatment and predicting the outcome. The concept of syndromes also has value in dispensing with the other parameters or assumptions

regarding the pathogenesis of epilepsy. Finally, the concept of epileptic syndromes is useful in research and comparative studies.

However, there are a number of potential deficiencies in the application of epileptic syndromes. First, epileptic syndromes do not provide any information as to the underlying etiology. West's syndrome, for example, may be due to a number of causes. Second, adherence to the criteria of any specific syndrome is essential; slipping an atypical case into a generally accepted syndrome is to be avoided as this defeats the whole objective of delineating and defining an epileptic syndrome.

Some syndromes have common signs and a predictable outcome, for example, benign rolandic epilepsy or benign occipital epilepsy. Others, such as absence seizures, are less specific and may include several subgroups with different outcomes and different associated features. Still others are, in fact, only loose collections of a few common characteristics inconstantly linked to one another.

The emphasis placed on epileptic syndromes is justified by the inadequacies and difficulties of the traditional approach to epilepsy, which is based on seizure types and the search for an underlying lesion. However, if the concept of epileptic syndromes is to be of any practical use, it has to be limited to those clusters that are unequivocally identifiable.

With the current advances in DNA and genetic studies, the idea of epileptic syndromes may eventually become redundant to be replaced by specific epileptic disorders. However, for the present, they serve to simplify the classification of epilepsy.

Classification of syndromes

Syndromic classification divides the epilepsies into two broad categories: localization-related and

Table 3.7 International League Against Epilepsy revised classification of epilepsy

(1) *Localization-related (focal, local, partial) epilepsies and syndromes*

    1.1   Idiopathic (with age-related onset)

          benign childhood epilepsy with centrotemporal spikes

          childhood epilepsy with occipital paroxysms

          primary reading epilepsy

    1.2   Symptomatic

          chronic progressive epilepsia partialis continua of childhood (Koshevnikoff's syndrome)

          syndromes characterized by seizures with specific modes of presentation

    1.3   Cryptogenic (presumed symptomatic but etiology unknown)

(2) *Generalized epilepsies and syndromes*

    2.1   Idiopathic (with age-related onset, listed in order of age)

          benign neonatal familial convulsions

          benign neonatal convulsions

          benign myoclonic epilepsy in infancy

          childhood absence epilepsy

          juvenile absence epilepsy

          juvenile myoclonic epilepsy

          epilepsy with grand mal (generalized tonic-clonic seizures) on awakening

          other generalized idiopathic epilepsies not defined above

          epilepsies with seizures precipitated by specific modes of activation (reflex and reading epilepsies)

    2.2   Cryptogenic or symptomatic (in order of age)

          West's syndrome

          Lennox–Gastaut syndrome

          epilepsy with myoclonic-astatic seizures

          epilepsy with myoclonic absences

    2.3   Symptomatic

        2.3.1 Non-specific etiology

             early myoclonic encephalopathy

             early infantile epileptic encephalopathy with suppression burst

             other symptomatic generalized epilepsies not defined above

        2.3.2 Specific syndromes / etiologies

             cerebral malformations

             inborn errors of metabolism including pyridoxine dependency and disorders frequently

                presenting as progressive myoclonic epilepsy

continued

(3) *Epilepsies and syndromes undetermined as to whether focal or generalized*

    3.1   With both generalized and focal seizures

        neonatal seizures

        severe myoclonic epilepsy in infancy

        epilepsy with continuous spike waves during slow-wave sleep

        acquired epileptic aphasia (Landau–Kleffner syndrome)

        other undetermined epilepsies not defined above

    3.2   Without unequivocal generalized or focal features

(4) *Special syndromes*

    4.1   Situation-related seizures

        febrile convulsions

        isolated seizures or isolated status epilepticus

        seizures occurring only when there is an acute metabolic or toxic event due to factors such as

            alcohol, drugs, eclampsia, non-ketotic hyperglycemia

        reflex epilepsy

From Commission on Classification and Terminology of the International League Against Epilepsy. Proposal for classification of epilepsies and epileptic syndromes. *Epilepsia* 1989;**30**:389–99

generalized. Each category is further subdivided into idiopathic, symptomatic and cryptogenic. Idiopathic epilepsies are age-related and have well-defined EEG characteristics whereas symptomatic/cryptogenic epilepsies occur at any age and have no typical EEG features. Four broad categories of epileptic syndrome are described.

Idiopathic generalized epilepsies commence in the first, second and third decades of life. Affected subjects have no associated intellectual or neurological deficits. These syndromes have a favorable prognosis with most patients responding to sodium valproate. The genetic bases of these syndromes have been well established and, although there is some overlap, twin studies indicate that specific syndromes are inherited within families.

Symptomatic generalized epilepsies are age-dependent encephalopathies characterized by onset in infancy/early childhood, and poor prognoses for both seizure control and development. Although these are distinct electroclinical entities, there is a degree of overlap. It is possible that these represent different responses to a wide range of insults at different stages of cerebral maturation.

Idiopathic partial epilepsies commence in childhood and include both the very commonly seen benign epilepsy of childhood with centrotemporal spikes and the relatively rare childhood epilepsy with occipital paroxysms. Both carry particularly benign prognoses.

Symptomatic partial epilepsies occur at any age with the most likely cause determined by the age of onset. Approximately 30% of cases of childhood epilepsy fall into this category. Adult-onset partial epilepsy is assumed to be symptomatic, although the cause often remains elusive.

Syndromic classification is less useful in these epilepsies where the most important consideration is definition of the cause which, in turn, determines the prognosis and influences management.

Examples of the commonly encountered age-related epileptic syndromes are shown in Figures 5–18.

Determination of cause

Epilepsy is a symptom not a diagnosis *per se*. An etiological classification of seizures and epilepsy is shown in Table 3.8.

Many cerebral pathologies may cause acute symptomatic seizures and, subsequently, epilepsy (Table 3.9). Acute symptomatic seizures may occur in response to a number of systemic disturbances (Table 3.10).

Unselected population-based studies indicate that the cause can be identified in approximately one-third of cases. The etiology may be inferred from the clinical history, which should include direct questioning on perinatal history and development, complicated early febrile convulsions (prolonged, focal or multiple episodes within 24 h), previous severe head injury, central nervous system infection, family history of epilepsy and the recent development of other neurological symptoms and signs.

Table 3.8 Classification of seizures and epilepsy by etiology

Acute symptomatic seizures

Isolated cryptogenic seizures

Epilepsies
   remote symptomatic
   genetic
   cryptogenic

Table 3.9 Central nervous system disease causing seizures and epilepsy

Congenital	hypoxic-ischemic cerebral insult birth trauma, tuberous sclerosis arteriovenous malformation lipid-storage diseases leukodystrophies Down syndrome
Infective	meningitis, encephalitis abscess, syphilis
Trauma	diffuse brain injury, hematoma (extradural, subdural, intracerebral) depressed skull fracture
Tumor	glioma, meningioma secondary carcinoma, etc.
Vascular	atheroma, arteritis, aneurysm
Degenerative	Alzheimer's, Batten's, Creutzfeldt–Jakob, Pick's diseases, etc.
Miscellaneous	demyelination

With permission from Chadwick D. Paroxysmal disorders. In: Chadwick D, Cartlidge NEF, Bates D, eds. *Medical Neurology*. Edinburgh: Churchill Livingstone, 1989:152–85

Table 3.10 Systemic disturbances causing seizures

Fever	Drugs
Hypoxia	Drug withdrawal
Hypoglycemia	Toxins
Electrolyte imbalance	
	Pyridoxine deficiency
Renal failure	Porphyria
Hepatic failure	Inborn errors of
Respiratory failure	metabolism

Age of onset is the most important indicator both of the likelihood of epilepsy being symptomatic and of the probable cause (Figure 18).

The principal role of EEG in epilepsy is in the classification of seizures / epilepsy. However, the presence of a focal slow- or spike-wave abnormality should raise the suspicion of a structural lesion and suggests the need for imaging.

There is no place for a policy of unselected computed tomography (CT) scanning in patients with epilepsy as clinically relevant abnormalities are rarely detected by this technology. However, CT is indicated in patients with later-onset partial seizures with or without neurological signs or focal EEG abnormalities, particularly in those who do not respond to treatment.

Magnetic resonance imaging (MRI) is superior to CT in the detection of small structural and subtle atrophic lesions, but is inferior to CT in demonstrating intracerebral calcification. In light of recent technological advances, MRI is now accepted as an essential part of presurgical investigation protocols, and is the imaging modality of choice when undertaking structural radiological investigation of patients (of all ages) with epilepsy. An independent role for functional imaging [single-photon emission computed tomography (SPECT) and positron emission tomography (PET)] remains undefined.

4 Etiology

Introduction

Epilepsy is a symptom, not a diagnosis, and not caused by a single disorder. Epilepsy may be due to virtually any cerebral pathology, and seizures may occur in association with a large number of systemic disorders. Although there are many causes of recurrent seizures and epilepsy, including cerebral hypoxia at birth, central nervous system infections, head trauma and brain tumors, no specific etiology can be found in almost two-thirds of patients.

This chapter reflects the heterogeneity of causes of epilepsy with an emphasis on clinicopathological correlations.

Perinatal causes

The newborn period is the time of life with the highest risk of seizures and epilepsy. The immature and developing brain is susceptible to a number of insults, including:

(1) *Asphyxia (hypoxic–ischemic encephalopathy).* This is the most common and also the most serious cause of neonatal seizures. Asphyxia usually occurs in term or postmature infants. The changes are those of necrosis of the deep cerebral white matter due to intrauterine or perinatal cerebral hypoxia, or ischemia.

Figures 19–22 illustrate the increasing severity of damage.

(2) *Intra- and periventricular hemorrhage* This phenomenon occurs predominantly in pre-term infants (Figures 23–26).

(3) *Transient metabolic dysfunction* This may occur, for example, in hypoglycemia, hypocalcemia or hyponatremia.

(4) *Sepsis* This may arise from congenital infections such as TORCH syndrome [*Toxoplasma* (Figures 27 and 28), other, rubella, cytomegalovirus (Figures 29–31) and herpes], and from syphilis, septicemia or meningitis.

(5) *Cerebral malformations / dysgenesis* These include hemimegalencephaly (Figures 32 and 33), lissencephaly (Figures 34 and 35), neuronal migration disorders (Figure 36), schizencephaly (Figure 37), Aicardi syndrome (Figure 38) with holoprosencephaly (Figures 39 and 40) and agenesis of the corpus callosum (Figures 41 and 42), lipoma of the corpus callosum (Figure 43), and temporal lobe agenesis (Figure 44).

It is the etiology of the seizures, rather than the seizures themselves, that is the predicting factor in the determination of 'late' epilepsy and intellectual status. The risk of late epilepsy is much greater if neonatal seizures were caused by hypoxic-ischemic encephalopathy or a cerebral malformation.

Neurodegenerative and metabolic encephalopathies

A number of rare age-related neurodegenerative conditions (Figure 45), including some inherited metabolic disorders, cause seizures and epilepsy. The clinical picture is usually progressive myoclonic epilepsy with or without dementia (Table 4.1).

Mitochondrial cytopathies

These form a heterogeneous group of multisystem diseases with diverse clinical presentations; the only common factor is a non-specific morphological finding on muscle biopsy – the 'ragged red' fiber (Figure

Table 4.1 Disorders in which clinical presentation is either typically or occasionally progressive myoclonic epilepsy

Typically progressive myoclonic epilepsy
Lafora's body disease
Ramsay Hunt syndrome
 (dyssynergia cerebellaris myoclonica)
Sialidosis type 1 (cherry-red spot myoclonus syndrome)
Sialidosis type 2
Mucolipidosis type 1
Juvenile neuropathic Gaucher's disease (type 3)
Juvenile neuroaxonal dystrophy

Occasionally progressive myoclonic epilepsy
Ceroid lipofuscinoses
 early and late infantile forms
 early and late juvenile forms
Myoclonic epilepsy with ragged red fibers (MERRF)
Huntington's disease
Wilson's disease
Hallervorden–Spatz disease

46). Myoclonic epilepsy with ragged red fibers (MERRF) usually presents in adolescence / early adulthood, but may occur at any age (Figure 47). Myoclonus, tonic-clonic seizures, muscle weakness and ataxia are prominent features. This phenotype is most frequently associated with maternal inheritance and has been linked to a point mutation of the transfer RNA lysine gene.

Lipidoses

These are a heterogeneous group of conditions characterized by accumulation of lipid-containing materials in neurons and other cells due to inherited lysosomal enzyme defects. A juvenile-onset form is characterized by extreme stimulus-sensitive myoclonus, generalized tonic-clonic seizures, dementia, rigidity, pseudobulbar palsy and, ultimately, quadriplegia. Rectal (Figure 48) and skin biopsies are useful methods of diagnosing lysosomal deficiency affecting the central nervous system.

Baltic myoclonus

This autosomal recessive condition has a peak age of onset at 10 years. The epilepsy is characterized by stimulus-sensitive myoclonus and generalized tonic-clonic seizures, both of which are usually well controlled with sodium valproate. Survival into adult life is common and the prognosis is much more favorable than previously recognized. Dementia does not occur, although phenytoin may be associated with a significant decline in cognitive function.

Lafora's body disease

This autosomal recessive condition is manifested by stimulus-sensitive myoclonus, generalized tonic-clonic seizures and partial seizures with visual auras. Onset is during childhood / adolescence. The clinical course involves progressive dementia, dysarthria and ataxia until death in the teens or early twenties. Pathologically, the condition is characterized by neuronal inclusions (Lafora's bodies; Figure 49) in the cerebellar cortex, brain stem nucleus and spinal cord.

Huntington's disease

This is characterized by the triad of dominant inheritance, choreoathetosis and progressive dementia. The responsible genetic defect is a trinucleotide expansion on the short arm of the fourth chromosome. The juvenile-onset form (Westphal variant) frequently presents with bradykinesia, rigidity and ataxia, and is associated with seizures in 50% of cases. The adult-onset form is occasionally complicated by a seizure disorder. The CT (Figure 50) and post-mortem findings (Figures 51 and 52) are striking.

Subacute spongiform encephalopathy (Creutzfeldt–Jakob disease)

This disease typically presents in middle age, but it may occur in young adults. In humans, transmission has been through corneal transplants, depth electrodes and human growth hormone injections. It is believed to be transmitted by a prion protein. After a latency period of 20–30 years (sometimes less), a rapidly progressive dementia ensues, culminating in death in less than a year. The EEG evolves into a characteristic pattern (Figure 53) and the histopathological features are also unique (Figure 54).

Alzheimer's disease

This is the most common of the neurodegenerative conditions. It usually commences in the seventh decade, although a familial, dominantly inherited, form occurs in mid-life. The onset is insidious and the course slowly progressive, with deterioration of memory, personality, language and, ultimately, motor function leading to death within 5–15 years. Alzheimer's disease is associated with a 10-fold increased risk of epilepsy compared with an age-matched population, and 15% experience seizures 10 years after diagnosis. Diffuse cerebral atrophy is visible on CT scanning (Figure 55) and the histological appearances are classical (Figures 56 and 57).

Reye's syndrome

This syndrome is a rare metabolic encephalopathy associated with the use of salicylic acid (aspirin), although a number of inborn errors of metabolism may also present with a picture resembling Reye's syndrome. Infants and young children present with repeated vomiting, fever, a disturbed conscious level and generalized convulsions. Most children have hypoglycemia and elevated concentrations of serum transaminases. There may be a prodromal viral illness, and different stages (or levels) of coma have been recognized. The mortality rate is high with death due (usually) to severe cerebral edema. The liver shows fatty infiltration, which resolves in survivors. Survivors also show varying degrees of neurological impairment and epilepsy (Figure 58).

Neurocutaneous syndromes

These constitute a collection of hereditary diseases caused by an unknown defect that affects structures of ectodermal origin. The syndromes are characterized by malformations and tumors in numerous organs, but notably in the skin, eye and nervous system. Three of the more common syndromes associated with epilepsy are described below.

Tuberous sclerosis This is transmitted as an autosomal dominant trait with incomplete penetrance which is strongly associated with male gender. The principal manifestations are mental retardation, seizures, skin lesions and tumors.

The classical cutaneous malformation is adenoma sebaceum (Figure 59). Additional cutaneous features include shagreen patches (Figure 60), periungual fibromata (Figure 61) and depigmented ash-leaf patches. The earliest sign may be a fibrous plaque on the forehead (Figure 62). Epilepsy is invariable in retarded patients and usual in the remainder. Tuberous sclerosis is a relatively common cause of infantile spasms; later presentation is in the form of partial or generalized seizures.

Benign cerebral, retinal (Figure 63) and renal tumors are found in 15%, 50% and 80% of cases, respectively. The tubers are areas of gliosis within the cerebral hemispheres in which extensive calcification results in a classical appearance on CT scanning (Figure 64). Additional cerebral dysgenesis is frequently seen in tuberous sclerosis (Figure 65) particularly with MRI.

Sturge–Weber syndrome (encephalotrigeminal angiomatosis) The full syndrome comprises a port-wine vascular nevus on the face, generalized or focal contralateral hemiparesis or homonymous hemianopia, ipsilateral intracranial calcification and mental retardation. The cutaneous angioma (Figure 66) is evident at birth and may extend to the pharynx or other viscera. Ninety per cent of cases develop seizures in the first year of life; hemiparesis occurs in 30–40% and mental retardation in 80%.

The leptomeningeal angiomatosis has a propensity for the occipital or occipitoparietal regions. Cortical calcification underlying the vascular malformation is evident on skull X-ray (Figure 67) and CT scanning (Figure 68).

Neurofibromatosis (NF) This dominantly inherited condition takes two forms: NF I (central) and NF II (peripheral). It is the most common single-gene defect affecting the central nervous system, with an incidence of 1 in 2000 population. Cutaneous lesions include café-au-lait spots (Figure 69), plexiform neurofibromata, axillary freckling and subcutaneous fibromata. Seizures occur in 10–15% of patients with NF I and are often associated with intracranial tumors (Figure 70).

Infections

Infections of the central nervous system account for 2–3% of all cases of epilepsy, but are among the most common causes in infants and preschool children. The risk of developing epilepsy and its subsequent prognosis depend on the severity of the illness and the age at which infection occurs.

Bacterial meningitis

The 20-year risk of later epilepsy is 13.4% if the acute illness is complicated by seizures and 2.4% if it is not. The apparently higher risk associated with certain organisms is probably due to their occurrence in younger children. Poor prognostic factors include extremes of age, bacteremia, seizures, coma, concomitant systemic illness and delayed treatment (Figures 71 and 72).

Cerebral abscess

Cerebral abscess is virtually always secondary to a suppurative process elsewhere in the body. The source may be within the skull (40%), metastatic (33%) or unidentified (20%). Effective antibiotic therapy and improvements in ear, nose and throat surgery have reduced the incidence of abscesses secondary to sinus or middle ear disease. The main sources of metastatic abscesses are from the heart (Figure 73) and lungs. Clinical presentation is variable with focal and generalized seizures being common. CT scanning is able to detect abscesses greater than 1 cm in diameter (Figure 74).

Initial treatment should be medical, with the choice of antibiotics guided by knowledge of the source of sepsis. Surgical intervention may be necessary if deterioration occurs. The advent of CT scanning has improved the prognosis, but the clinical course remains unpredictable and the mortality rate is still approximately 20% (Figure 75). Focal epilepsy is the most common sequela and the risk rises over time.

On 10-year follow-up, 90% of the patients requiring surgical intervention will have developed this complication.

Subdural empyema

This usually occurs as a consequence of frontal or ethmoidal sinusitis (Figure 76) due to direct extension or venous spread of infection. The most common offending pathogens are streptococci.

Focal seizures, due to local cerebral ischemic necrosis, are a late feature associated with a rapidly deteriorating conscious level. CT scanning is diagnostic (Figure 77). Urgent surgical drainage is usually required, but the mortality rate is high (Figure 78).

Herpes simplex encephalitis

This is the most common and most severe form of acute encephalitis. Acute symptomatic seizures and symptoms suggesting temporal lobe involvement are common presenting features. Cerebrospinal fluid lymphocytosis is usual, but a high red-cell count and xanthochromia reflect the hemorrhagic nature of the lesions. The EEG (Figure 79) has a typical appearance, but this is not specific to herpes simplex encephalitis. In children, the classical EEG appearances may not be seen (Figure 80).

CT scanning will confirm temporal lobe damage (Figure 81) and may be useful in differentiating herpes simplex encephalitis from other causes of coma with fever.

Cerebral biopsy (Figure 82) is rarely indicated as intravenous acyclovir should be initiated as soon as the diagnosis is suspected.

The risk of mortality depends on the age and the level of consciousness at the time of institution of antiviral therapy. Intense hemorrhagic necrosis of the temporal lobe is seen at necropsy (Figure 83).

In survivors, neurological sequelae are almost inevitable, the most common of which are amnesic syndromes, dysphasia and temporal lobe epilepsy. The 20-year risk of epilepsy is twice as great if acute symptomatic seizures occur (22% vs 10%), which is higher than after bacterial meningitis presumably because of direct cerebral parenchymal damage.

HIV and Toxoplasma infection

Human immunodeficiency virus (HIV) infection and the acquired immune deficiency syndrome (AIDS) have reached pandemic proportions. Neurological manifestations are commonly seen and may be due to direct viral invasion or be secondary to immunosuppression. Seizures occur in 10–20% of unselected populations of patients with HIV infection. These are generalized in 75% of cases, but partial-onset seizures may occur in the absence of focal structural pathology. Both convulsive and non-convulsive status have been reported. Of those with seizures, 15% are seropositive only, 15% have AIDS-related complex and 70% have full-blown AIDS.

Generalized seizures are a common late feature of the AIDS–dementia complex, probably due to progressive cortical damage. Convulsive status, which is associated with a poor prognosis, may simply reflect late severe AIDS. The EEG is usually abnormal, but specific epileptiform features are unusual and, with the exception of non-convulsive status, the EEG rarely yields additional useful clinical information.

Cerebral HIV infection (Figure 84) and secondary neoplastic or infective conditions (Figures 85–88) are responsible for the seizures in roughly equal proportions. Of the opportunistic infections with a predilection for the central nervous system, the protozoon Toxoplasma gondii is the most frequently implicated. Cerebral toxoplasma infection usually presents as meningoencephalitis, although an encephalopathic picture may occur. Seizures are seen in 30% of cases.

The diagnosis is confirmed by positive serology, cerebrospinal fluid culture and CT appearances (Figure 89). Differentiation from the direct effects of HIV infection is important as this is a treatable complication. As it represents a reactivation of pre-existing infection, treatment with sulfadiazine and pyrimethamine has to be lifelong. The condition is fatal if allowed to continue unrecognized; *Toxoplasma* abscesses (Figures 90–92) were found in 13% of one reported AIDS autopsy series.

Neurocysticercosis

Cysticercosis is the larval stage of infection by the pork tapeworm *Taenia solium*. In both Central and South America, it is the leading cause of epilepsy and other neurological disorders. Other cerebral manifestations include obstructive hydrocephalus, focal deficits and, rarely, subarachnoid hemorrhages. Tonic-clonic seizures are the most common presenting feature. Early treatment with praziquantel abolishes the need for continuing antiepileptic drugs in 70% of cases but, if the lesions calcify (Figure 93), a permanent epileptogenic focus may result. The radiographic appearances may be more florid in the untreated patient (Figure 94).

Cerebral malaria

Cerebral malaria complicates 2% of infections with falciparum malaria. Children, pregnancy, immunosuppression and cessation of antimalarial prophylaxis increase the risk. A rapidly fatal encephalopathy usually occurs during the second or third week of the illness, but may also be the initial presentation. The appearances on necropsy are characteristic (Figure 95).

Tuberculosis

Tuberculous meningitis is rare in developed countries, but remains a common problem among the underdeveloped countries. The usual presentation is an insidious meningoencephalitis. Other complications include cranial nerve palsies, cerebral infarction and obstructive hydrocephalus. Tuberculomas (Figure 96) account for 5–30% of intracranial mass lesions reported in underdeveloped countries, and may present with focal seizures and signs (Figure 97).

Subacute sclerosing panencephalitis

This extremely rare subacute or chronic encephalopathy usually affects children and young adults. It typically presents 6–10 years after primary measles infection and may represent an abnormal immune response. The inexorable course is characterized by dementia, myoclonus, seizures, ataxia, rigidity and death usually, but not invariably, within 1–3 years. The diagnosis is confirmed by the classical EEG and MRI appearances (Figures 98 and 99), elevated IgG concentrations in the cerebrospinal fluid, and raised measles antibody titers in the serum and cerebrospinal fluid. The postmortem findings are pathognomonic (Figures 100 and 101).

Neurosyphilis

Untreated infection with *Treponema pallidum* may affect the central nervous system after a variable (1–30 years) period of latency. Neurosyphilis is classified as tertiary (meningovascular) or quarternary (parenchymatous). The latter involves direct treponemal invasion of the neurons of the cerebrum (general paresis of the insane) or the spinal cord (tabes dorsalis).

General paresis of the insane presents with insidious mental changes and gradually progresses to a profound dementia. Seizures, either localized or generalized, occur in 50% of cases and may be the presenting symptom whereas focal deficits are a late feature. There is usually a cerebrospinal fluid pleocytosis. Specific treponemal tests indicate previous infection and remain positive throughout life, but may be negative with concomitant HIV infections. Non-specific lipoidal tests provide an index of disease activity. The diagnosis requires a high degree of suspicion as early treatment may be effective. However, the prognosis is generally poor with death ensuing within 2–5 years (Figures 102 and 103).

Rasmussen's 'encephalitis'

This rare syndrome usually develops during early to mid-childhood and is characterized by either a gradual or an explosive onset of frequent focal seizures, including epilepsia partialis continua. Progressive hemiplegia and other neurological deficits develop, and death may follow either rapidly or after a period of apparent stabilization. CT or MRI of the affected hemisphere will show progressive atrophy and PET will reveal hypometabolism.

The etiology of the syndrome is unknown, although a low-grade viral infection (possibly with cytomegalovirus) has been implicated. However, the causes may be multiple (Figures 104–106).

The seizures are resistant to most antiepileptic drugs. Corticosteroids and other immunosuppressants have been used with variable success, as has surgery (usually hemispherectomy).

Genetic epilepsies

Genetic factors may be implicated in up to 50% of all epilepsies. Many inherited disorders are manifested by seizures and several specific epilepsy syndromes have a predominantly genetic basis. Recent developments have helped to clarify the complex relationships between seizures / epilepsy and heredity. These relationships are likely to have diagnostic, prognostic and, ultimately, therapeutic implications.

Hereditary disorders and epilepsy

A total of 160 Mendelian traits (single-gene defects) are associated with seizures with or without mental retardation. Autosomal recessive traits, which are often due to enzyme defects, are the most likely to manifest seizures (Table 4.2).

Multifactorial (polygenic) and maternally inherited conditions are also well documented. Examples of the conditions associated with each mode of inheritance are shown in Table 4.3.

The risks of epilepsy occurring in patients with some chromosomal abnormalities are presented in Table 4.4.

Table 4.2 Mendelian traits associated with seizures, with and without mental retardation

	Total (n)	Seizures and retardation		Seizures only		Total seizures	
		n	%	n	%	n	%
Autosomal dominant	3047	19	0.6	24	0.8	43	1.4
Autosomal recessive	1554	79	5.1	19	1.2	98	6.3
X-linked recessive	336	15	4.5	4	1.2	19	5.7
Total	4937	113	2.3	47	1.0	160	3.2

From McKusick VA. *Mendelian Inheritance in Man*, 9th edn. Baltimore: Johns Hopkins University Press, 1990

Table 4.3 Hereditary disorders leading to conditions associated with seizures by mode of inheritance

Mode of inheritance	Condition
Mendelian (symptomatic)	
Autosomal recessive	Unverricht–Lundborg disease infantile NCL juvenile NCL (Batten diease) Lafora's body disease Northern epilepsy
Autosomal dominant	tuberous sclerosis complex neurofibromatosis type I Miller–Dieker syndrome
X-linked	fragile X syndrome band heterotopia / lissencephaly periventricular nodular heterotopia
Mendelian (idiopathic)	

Autosomal dominant (AD)	benign familial neonatal
	  convulsions
	benign familial infantile
	  convulsions
	(AD) nocturnal frontal lobe
	  epilepsy
	(AD) partial epilepsies:
	  with auditory symptoms
	  with speech dyspraxia
	  with variable foci
	  with temporal lobe epilepsy

Non-Mendelian (idiopathic)	
Complex inheritance	juvenile myoclonic epilepsy childhood absence epilepsy benign childhood epilepsy with centrotemporal spikes
Maternal inheritance mitochondrial DNA mutations	MELAS, MERRF

NCL, neuronal ceroid lipofuscinosis; MELAS, mitochondrial encephalopathy, lactic acidosis and strokes; MERRF, myoclonic epilepsy with ragged red fibers

Table 4.4 Risks of epilepsy in patients with specific chromosomal disorders

Condition	Risk of epilepsy
Down syndrome	5.8–10.2% of hospitalized patients
Ring C14	6 / 7 myoclonus + GTCS
Inverted duplicated C15	21 / 28 reported cases
Ring C20	7 / 12 CPS + SGTCS
Fragile X syndrome	common
Angelman's syndrome	all

C14, C15, C20, chromosomes 14, 15, 20; GTCS, generalized tonic-clonic seizure; CPS, complex partial seizure; SGTCS, secondary generalized tonic-clonic seizure

Angelman's syndrome

This is a rare disorder that affects children, comprising psychomotor and profound speech and language delay, epilepsy (commonly myoclonic and tonic-atonic seizures) and an abnormal effect characterized by almost continuous smiling and episodes of inappropriate laughter. Because of these latter features and the child's frequent jerky movements, the condition is also known as the 'happy puppet' syndrome. The EEG may be helpful in establishing the diagnosis (Figure 107). The condition has a genetic basis, with most children having an abnormality of chromosome 15.

Rett syndrome

This is a rare syndrome of unknown cause which affects girls only, and is seen with a frequency of 1 / 10 000–15 000. The condition is characterized by developmental regression, acquired microcephaly, epilepsy, episodes of hyperventilation and repetitive stereotypical hand-wringing movements. The epilepsy usually begins after the age of 2 years and includes tonic, atonic, myoclonic and atypical absence seizures. The EEG may be helpful in establishing the diagnosis (Figure 108).

Genetics of epilepsy syndromes

Whereas the relatives of patients with partial-onset seizures have only a slightly increased risk of developing epilepsy, recent research has identified several dominantly inherited conditions (see Table 4.3). The genetic basis of the idiopathic epilepsies, with their characteristic generalized spike-and-wave patterns on EEG, is well established. There is some degree of overlap (Figure 109), and twin studies indicate that specific syndromes are inherited within families. This knowledge has implications for patient counselling. Although a positive family history of a seizure disorder may be obtained in up to 40% of patients with childhood absence or juvenile myoclonic epilepsy, the risk to their siblings is relatively low (Figure 110).

Recently, the genetic loci of three epilepsy syndromes have been mapped to specific chromosomes (Figures 111 and 112). While juvenile myoclonic epilepsy was originally linked to chromosome 6, recent evidence suggests that this clinical phenotype is genetically heterogeneous. The most likely gene defects are those involving the ion channels and membrane receptors. Indeed, a mutation of the neuronal nicotinic acetylcholine receptor gene has been identified in autosomal-dominant nocturnal frontal lobe epilepsy.

At present, the implications of this information are mainly for counselling and reassurance. However, if the metabolic defects coded by the relevant genes can be identified, this may permit the development of syndrome-specific treatment.

Head injuries

The relationship between head injury, acute symptomatic seizures and late post-traumatic epilepsy is well documented. The risk of post-traumatic epilepsy is directly related to the severity of the cerebral insult.

Penetrating head injury

Penetrating head wounds resulting from missile injuries carry a 50% risk of post-traumatic epilepsy. Factors increasing the risk include involvement of the motor-premotor cortex, extent of cerebral tissue loss and, particularly, the development of abscess formation. This type of injury carries the highest relative risk of developing epilepsy of any cerebral insult (Figure 113). On 15-year follow-up, more than 50% of patients have active epilepsy.

Blunt trauma

The risks of early seizures (within 1 week) and post-traumatic epilepsy in an unselected population of patients with blunt head trauma (Table 4.5) are clearly related to the severity of the insult (Table 4.6). The relative risk of such patients developing epilepsy falls over time (12.7 at 1 year, 4.4 at 1–5 years and 1.4 after 5 years). Table 4.7 shows the definitions of mild, moderate and severe head injury.

Table 4.5 Risk of early seizures following blunt head trauma

	Adults (%)	Children (%)
Overall	1.8	2.8
Severe head injury	10.3	30.5

Table 4.6 Risk of late epilepsy following blunt head trauma according to severity of injury

Severity	1 year (%)	5 years (%)
Severe	7.1	11.5
Moderate	0.7	1.6
Mild	0.1	0.6

In a selected population referred to a neurological center, 5% of survivors developed post-traumatic epilepsy. Significant risk factors (Table 4.8) included early seizures, depressed skull fracture with dural laceration (Figure 114) and intracranial hematoma (Figures 115 and 116).

On 15-year follow-up, 50% of patients will be in a 5-year remission of seizures whereas 25% will experience more than six seizures per year. Despite the ability to predict which patients have a high risk of developing post-traumatic epilepsy, prospective controlled studies have failed to demonstrate any benefit of prophylactic antiepileptic agents.

Cerebral tumors

Primary intracranial neoplasms are rare. It is now generally accepted that they arise *de novo* as a result of neoplastic transformation of elements in adults. Environmental factors are probably of etiological importance but, apart from radiation, no specific factor has been implicated.

Seizures are a common presentation of primary cerebral tumors, but tumors are a relatively rare cause of epilepsy especially in children. In the National General Practice Study of Epilepsy[1], a tumor was identified in 6% of all new cases (Figure 117), but accounted for 19% of cases involving patients aged 40–59 years. The diagnosis should be suspected in patients with late-onset partial epilepsy especially if there are focal signs, focal slow waves on the EEG or a poor initial response to treatment.

Presentation with epilepsy is a favorable prognostic factor (Figure 118) in patients with tumors, and may be the only manifestation for years, reflecting a relatively benign underlying pathology. Indeed, although low-grade astrocytomas and oligodendrogliomas are complicated by epilepsy in 60–90% of cases, malignant gliomas usually present with progressive focal deficits.

Table 4.7 Definitions of mild, moderate and severe head injury

Degree	Definition
Severe	brain contusion, intracerebral or intracranial hematoma, or 24 h of unconsciousness or amnesia
Moderate	skull fracture, or 30 min–24 h of unconsciousness or post-traumatic amnesia
Mild	Briefer periods of unconsciousness or amnesia

Table 4.8 Risk factors for post-traumatic epilepsy

Risk factor	Incidence (%)
Intracranial hematoma	33
Early seizures	25
Depressed skull fracture	24*

*The risk is doubled if post-traumatic amnesia lasts > 24 h

A number of other clinical and CT features are useful as prognostic indicators (Table 4.9). Although aggressive management improves survival in cases with highly malignant tumors, such an approach is not of proven value in cases of slow-growing lesions presenting with epilepsy (Table 4.10).

Tumor-associated epilepsy is particularly resistant to antiepileptic drugs and the outcome of surgery depends on the resectability of the lesion.

Glioblastoma multiforme

This highly malignant astrocytic tumor is the most common glioma affecting the cerebral hemispheres in adults. Seizures occur in 30–40% of patients, but focal signs and enhancing lesions on CT scanning

Table 4.9 Relative risk (RR) of mortality associated with different variables (whole study population) using Cox's stepwise proportional hazards model

	Beta	p	RR (95% CI)
Age	0.0218	< 0.0001	
First symptom of epilepsy	-0.7815	< 0.0001	0.46 (0.34, 0.61)
Deep x-ray therapy	-0.7849	< 0.0001	0.46 (0.36, 0.57)
Non-resective surgery	0.5666	< 0.0001	1.76 (1.43, 2.17)
Focal signs	0.4483	0.0001	1.56 (1.24, 1.97)
Enhancement on CT	0.3999	0.0018	1.49 (1.16, 1.92)
Cyst on CT	-0.2822	0.0124	0.75 (0.60, 0.94)

Table 4.10 Relative risk (RR) of mortality associated with different variables (first symptom of epilepsy) using Cox's stepwise proportional hazards model

	Beta	p	RR (95% CI)
Focal signs	1.0972	< 0.0001	3.0 (1.86, 4.81)
Age	0.0425	< 0.0001	
Enhancement on CT	1.0044	0.0001	2.73 (1.65, 3.79)
Non-resective surgery	0.8790	0.0002	2.45 (1.52, 3.82)
Gender	0.4571	0.0474	1.58 (1.01, 2.56)

(Figure 119) are usually found at presentation. These lesions are large and frequently involve both hemispheres (Figure 120). The histological appearances are characteristic (Figure 121).

Low-grade astrocytoma

These relatively benign tumors often cause refractory partial epilepsy in neurologically intact patients. The initial CT scan usually shows a non-enhancing low-density lesion (Figure 122). With time, neurological deficits develop and the CT appearances indicate increased tumor activity.

These slow-growing lesions are diffusely infiltrative (Figure 123) and rarely amenable to complete surgical excision. The histological appearances are typical (Figure 124).

Oligodendroglioma

These tumors account for less than 10% of all gliomas and are seen more frequently in male patients. Calcification (Figure 125) occurs in more than 50% of lesions, probably as a reflection of their slow growth rate, and is also visible on CT scanning (Figure 126).

Surgery and radiotherapy are of no proven benefit in the management of these patients. However, these lesions may sometimes regress with chemotherapy using the nitrogen mustards (N,N-bis(2-chloroethyl)-N-nitrosourea and N-(2-chloroethyl)-N'-cyclohexyl-N-nitrosourea).

Meningioma

These benign tumors usually arise from arachnoid cells, but may be derived from dural fibroblasts. They comprise 15% of intracranial tumors and are more commonly seen in women. Peak onset is in the seventh decade, but they may occur earlier in patients with a history of deep X-ray therapy to the scalp or cranium.

The sylvian regions are a site of predilection, and presentation with focal seizures is common. Erosion of the overlying bone is often seen on CT scanning

(Figure 127). Accessible surface lesions should be excised (Figure 128), but recurrence is possible if excision is not complete. Benign histological features are typical (Figure 129).

Cerebral secondaries

Metastatic carcinoma is much more common than primary intracranial tumors. The most common primary sites, in order of frequency, are the lung, breast, skin (melanoma), colon and kidney. The lung and breast alone account for 50% of cerebral metastases. On CT scanning and on radiology, lesions usually appear to be solid and well circumscribed with marked local edema (Figures 130–132). Metastases are frequently multiple.

Primary cerebral lymphoma

This tumor corresponds to the histiocytic type of malignant lymphoma in the Rappaport classification system. It is rare, but the incidence is increasing. Patients with AIDS and long-term immunosuppression, especially renal-transplant patients, are at particular risk. In patients who are not immunosuppressed, there is some evidence that the Epstein–Barr virus may be causative.

The clinical presentation is similar to that of malignant gliomas but, on CT, the appearances may be strikingly different (Figure 133).

There may be dramatic clinical and radiological improvement after treatment with steroids (Figure 134), but this positive response is only temporary with a median survival of 24 months. Postmortem examination reveals the malignant features of these lesions (Figures 135 and 136).

Cerebrovascular disease

In the National General Practice Study of Epilepsy[1], a large community-based study, there was evidence

Table 4.11 Non-malignant neurosurgical conditions and incidence of seizures

Condition	Incidence of seizures (%)
Vascular	
anterior cerebral artery aneurysm	21
middle cerebral artery aneurysm	38
arteriovenous malformation	50
spontaneous hematoma	20
Meningioma	22
Abscess	92
Other benign supratentorial tumors	4
Shunting for hydrocephalus	17

With permission, from Foy PM, Copeland GP, Shaw MDM. The incidence of post-operative seizures. *Acta Neurochir* 1981;**55**:253–64

of cerebrovascular disease in 15% of patients with newly diagnosed epilepsy. This is the most common cause of epilepsy in the elderly, accounting for up to one-third of cases.

Hemorrhagic strokes carry a much greater risk of epilepsy than do ischemic events (Figure 137). The 1-year risk after a subarachnoid hemorrhage is 20%, but this increases after a middle cerebral artery aneurysm has been clipped (see below). The incidence is even greater in patients with arteriovenous malformation, especially if they have bled or been treated surgically (Table 4.11).

Cerebral infarction

This probably accounts for one-third of all cases of epilepsy commencing after 60 years of age (Figures 138–140). A recent retrospective population-based study reported risks of early (less than 1 week) and late (more than 1 week) seizures to be 6.2% and 7.4%, respectively. Early seizures often occur within 24 h. Infarction in the anterior cerebral hemispheres and embolic events carry higher risks. Of the cases with late seizures, 73% occurred within 2 years of stroke.

Middle cerebral artery aneurysm

Unruptured aneurysms rarely cause seizures, but there is a high risk of epilepsy if they bleed and, in particular, after surgical treatment of a middle cerebral artery aneurysm (Figure 141).

Arteriovenous malformations

These are developmental anomalies which involve abnormal communications between the arterial and venous systems (Figures 142 and 143). The most common presentations are subarachnoid hemorrhage, epilepsy, chronic headache and, rarely, progressive neurological deficit. If untreated, the cumulative risk of hemorrhage is 1–2% per annum.

Of these lesions, 20–40% are amenable to surgery, but the operative morbidity is high and the risk of epilepsy is increased. Embolization is reserved for lesions with a single large feeding vessel whereas stereotactic radiotherapy can obliterate smaller lesions.

Venous sinus thrombosis

Occlusion of the cerebral venous sinuses is an uncommon cause of stroke. Most cases are idiopathic, but predisposing factors include local sepsis, disseminated malignancy, hypercoagulability states and the puerperium.

The primary pathological event is cerebral infarction, but hemorrhage often supervenes. Clinical features vary according to the site of venous occlusion, with hemiplegia and seizures being a common presentation of sagittal-sinus thrombosis. Diagnosis may be suspected on CT (Figure 144) and can be confirmed by angiography or non-invasively by MRI (Figure 145).

The overall mortality is 20–30% and is dependent on the underlying cause. The efficacy of heparinization requires confirmation by a large-scale controlled clinical trial. The incidence of late epilepsy is not known.

Intracerebral hematoma

This is usually the consequence of moderate-to-severe hypertension. Hemorrhage is classified as massive, small or slit, with the prognosis directly related to size. Sites of predilection include the putamen, thalamus, pons, cerebellum and lobes. Patients with lobar hemorrhage (Figure 146) are more usually normotensive and an underlying arteriovenous malformation should be suspected. Seizures occur in 10–20% of cases.

Cerebral lupus

Systemic lupus erythematosus commonly involves the central nervous system. The cerebral manifestations are caused by widespread microinfarction due to arteriolar proliferation and destruction rather than by true vasculitis.

The clinical manifestations are protean, but seizures, cognitive and behavioral symptoms, and focal signs predominate. The cerebrospinal fluid and CT scan are often normal, and MRI is the investigation of choice. Discrete and diffuse patterns of magnetic resonance abnormality can be identified, with the latter more commonly associated with seizures (Figure 147).

Seizures and epilepsy following cardiac bypass surgery

Cardiopulmonary bypass surgery has increased in both sophistication and availability over the past decade. Total correction of previously inoperable congenital cardiac defects is being undertaken at progressively younger ages, and coronary artery and valve replacement is being performed in adults with increasing frequency.

Although most patients undergo surgery without complications, neurological sequelae may occur as a consequence of microembolization, hypoxia, cerebral hypoperfusion (ischemia) and metabolic dysfunction. Seizures are a common complication and may be either transient or persistent. Patients may develop both focal and generalized epileptic seizures. Focal seizures are often difficult to control and are refractory to antiepileptic drug treatment (Figure 148). Chronic epilepsy in these situations is frequently associated with neurological deficit and cognitive dysfunction.

Reference

1. Sander JWAS, Hart YM, Johnson AL, Shorvon SD. National General Practice Study of Epilepsy: Newly diagnosed epileptic seizures in a general population. *Lancet* 1990;**336**:1267–71.

5 Prognosis

Epilepsy

Prior to the availability of effective antiepileptic drugs, epilepsy was probably a chronic disabling condition in most cases. Even after the discovery of effective antiepileptic drugs, selected hospital-based statistics suggested a poor prognosis, with only approximately 30% of patients achieving remission (Table 5.1).

In contrast, recent studies (Table 5.2) in unselected populations have demonstrated a favorable outlook with up to 70% of patients achieving protracted remission (Figure 149).

Although the overall prognosis is good, 25–30% of patients continue to have seizures despite optimal drug therapy. This reflects the heterogeneity of the epilepsies and several biological variables that influ-

Table 5.1 Prognostic studies of chronic epilepsy

Reference	n	Duration of remission (years)	Percentage in remission
Habermass (1901)	937	2	10
Turner (1907)	87	2	32
Grosz (1930)	125	10	11
Kirstein (1942)	174	3	22
Alstroem (1950)	897	5	22
Strobos (1959)	228	1	38
Kjorbe, Lund & Poulsen (1960)	130	4	32
Probst (1960)	83	2	31
Trolle (1960)	799	2	37
Juul-Jensen (1963)	969	2	32
Lorge (1964)	177	2	34

With permission, from Reynolds EH. The prognosis of epilepsy: Is chronic epilepsy preventable? In: Trimble MR, ed. *Chronic Epilepsy, its Prognosis and Management.* Chichester: John Wiley & Sons, 1989:13–20[1]

Table 5.2 Prognostic studies in newly diagnosed patients

Reference	n	Duration of remission (years)	Percentage in remission
Annegers, Hauser & Elveback, 1979[2]	457	5	70.0
Okuma & Kumashiro, 1981[3]	1868	4	69.0
Goodridge & Shorvon, 1983[4]	122	3	58.3
Elwes et al., 1984[5]	106	2	82.0
Collaborative Group, 1992[6]*	283	2	67.5

*This study included 51 patients with isolated seizures

Table 5.3 Adverse prognostic factors

Symptomatic etiology

Partial-onset seizures

Atonic seizures

Late-onset or first-year epilepsy

Additional mental or motor handicap

Long duration prior to treatment

Poor initial response to treatment

Table 5.4 Prognosis by epilepsy syndrome

Good
Benign neonatal familial convulsions
Childhood absence epilepsy
Benign childhood epilepsy with rolandic spikes
Juvenile myoclonic epilepsy (but relapses common
    if treatment discontinued)
Epilepsy with grand mal on awakening

Intermediate
Benign myoclonic epilepsy of infancy
Juvenile absence epilepsy
Myoclonic–astatic epilepsy

Poor
Ohtahara syndrome (early infantile epileptic
    encephalopathy)
West's syndrome
Lennox–Gastaut syndrome

Table 5.5 Prognostic variables for recurrence after antiepileptic drug withdrawal

Variable	RR	95% CI
Period seizure-free		
< 2.5 years	1.00	
2.5–< 3 years	0.94	0.67, 1.32
3–< 5 years	0.67	0.48, 0.93*
5–< 10 years	0.47	0.32, 0.69*
History of partial seizures only	2.51	1.00, 6.30†
History of myoclonic seizures	1.85	1.09, 3.12†
History of tonic-clonic seizures	3.40	1.48, 7.84†
More than one antiepileptic drug at randomization	1.79	1.34, 2.39†
Seizures after start of treatment	1.57	1.10, 2.24†

RR, relative risk
Adapted with permission, from reference 7
*Factors associated with lower risk of relapse
†Factors associated with higher risk of relapse

ence the prognosis in a given patient. Studies in unselected populations consistently identify a limited number of interdependent variables (Table 5.3) which characterize patients likely to develop a chronic condition. The prognosis of any patient with epilepsy is dependent on the underlying syndrome (Table 5.4) and/or its cause.

Table 5.6 Prognosis for recurrence after 'first' seizures

Reference	n	Median follow-up	Time at which outcome was ascertained	Recurrence risk (%)
First-seizure methods				
Prospective ascertainment				
Hauser et al., 1990[8]	208	> 2 years	5 years	34
Shinnar et al., 1991[9]	283	2.7 years	4 years	42
Camfield et al., 1989[10]	47	1 year	1 year	38
Hopkins et al., 1988[11]	306	—	4 years	52
Pearce & Mackintosh, 1979[12]	22	>12 months	1 year	23
Retrospective ascertainment				
Boulloche et al., 1989[13]	119	> 5 years	8 years	38
Annegers et al., 1986[14]	424	> 2 years	5 years	56
Camfield et al., 1985[15]	168	2 years	2 years	52
Elwes et al., 1985[16]	133	15 months	3 years	71
Cleland et al., 1981[17]	70	4 years	—	39
Hyllested & Pakkenberg, 1963[18]	63	> 4 years	—	43
Thomas, 1959[19]	48	> 3 years	—	27
Saunders & Marshal, 1975[20]	39	2 years	—	33
New-onset epilepsy methods				
Prospective ascertainment				
Blom et al., 1978[21]	74	3 years	3 years	58
Retrospective ascertainment				
Hertz et al., 1984[22]	435	to age 7	at age 7	69
van den Berg & Yerushally, 1969[23]	113	to age 5	at age 5	65

With permission, from Berg AT, Shinnar S. The risk of recurrence following a first unprovoked seizure. *Neurology* 1991;41:965-72

Drug withdrawal

In a heterogeneous group of patients with epilepsy in remission, planned withdrawal of antiepileptic drugs doubled the risk of relapse at 2 years (Figure 150). Multivariate analysis demonstrated a limited number of independently significant prognostic variables (Table 5.5). From these data, a predictive model has been developed from which a patient's risk of relapse at 1 and 2 years can be calculated.

Single seizures

Methodological differences explain the widely varying estimates of the risk of recurrence after an isolated seizure (Table 5.6). Meta-analysis of prospective studies, using first-seizure methods, indicates an overall 2-year risk of 30–40%.

Etiology and the EEG appear to be the most important predictors of recurrence. When these factors are combined, the lowest risk (24%) is in the idiopathic group with a normal EEG, and the highest risk (65%) is in remote symptomatic seizures associated with an epileptiform EEG.

The influence of treatment on recurrence is not known. An ongoing prospective randomized study of treatment vs observation in early epilepsy and single seizures [MRC Study of Epilepsy and Single Seizures (MESS)] should clarify this issue.

References

1. Reynolds EH. The prognosis of epilepsy: Is chronic epilepsy preventable? In: Trimble MR, ed. *Chronic Epilepsy, its Prognosis and Management.* Chichester: John Wiley & Sons, 1989:13–20

2. Annegers JF, Hauser WA, Elveback LR. Remission of seizures and relapse in patients with epilepsy. *Epilepsia* 1979;**20**:729–37

3. Okuma T, Kumashiro H. Natural history and prognosis of epilepsy: Report of a multi-institutional study in Japan. *Epilepsia* 1981;**22**:25–53

4. Goodridge DMG, Shorvon SD. Epileptic seizures in a population of 6,000. II. Treatment and prognosis. *BMJ* 1983;**287**:645–7

5. Elwes RDC, Johnson AL, Shorvon SD, Reynolds EH. The prognosis for seizure control in newly diagnosed epilepsy. *N Engl J Med* 1984;**311**:944–7

6. Collaborative Group for the Study of Epilepsy. Prognosis of epilepsy in newly referred patients: A multicentre study of the effects of monotherapy on the long-term course of epilepsy. *Epilepsia* 1992;**33**:45–51

7. MRC Antiepileptic Drug Withdrawal Study Group. A randomized study of anti-epileptic drug withdrawal in patients in remission of epilepsy. *Lancet* 1991;**i**:1175–80

8. Hauser WA, Rich SS, Annegers JF, Anderson VE. Seizure recurrence after a first unprovoked seizure: An extended follow-up. *Neurology* 1990;**40**:1163–70

9. Shinnar S, Berg AT, Moshe SL, et al. The risk of recurrence following a first unprovoked seizure in childhood: A prospective study. *Pediatrics* 1991;**85**:1076–85

10. Camfield P, Camfield C, Dooley A, Smith E, Garner B. A randomized study of carbamazepine versus no medication after a first unprovoked seizure in childhood. *Neurology* 1989;**39**:851–2

11. Hopkins A, Garman A, Clark C. The first seizure in adult life: Value of clinical features, electroencephalography and computerised tomographic scanning in prediction of seizure recurrence. *Lancet* 1988;**i**:721–6

12. Pearce JL, Mackintosh HT. Prospective study of convulsions in childhood. *NZ Med J* 1979;**89**: 1–3

13. Boulloche I, Leloup P, Mallet E, Parain D, Tron P. Risk of recurrence after a single unprovoked generalised tonic-clonic seizure. *Dev Med Child Neurol* 1989;**39**:626–32

14. Annegers JF, Shirts SB, Hauser WA, Kurland LT. The risk of recurrence after an initial unprovoked seizure. *Epilepsia* 1986;**27**:43–50

15. Camfield PR, Camfield CS, Dooley JM, Tibbles JAR, Fung T, Garner B. Epilepsy after a first unprovoked seizure in childhood. *Neurology* 1985;**35**:1657–60

16. Elwes RDC, Chesterman P, Reynolds EH. Prognosis after a first untreated tonic-clonic seizure. *Lancet* 1985;**ii**:752–3

17. Cleland PG, Mosquera I, Stuard WP, Foster JB. Prognosis of isolated seizures in adult life. *Lancet* 1981;**ii**:1364

18. Hyllested K, Pakkenberg H. Prognosis in epilepsy of late onset. *Neurology* 1963;**13**:641–4

19. Thomas MH. The single seizure – its study and management. *J Am Med Assoc* 1959;**169**:457–9

20. Saunders M, Marshal C. Isolated seizures: An EEG and clinical assessment. *Epilepsia* 1975;**16**: 731–3

21. Blom S, Heijbel J, Bergfors PG. Incidence of epilepsy in children: A follow-up study three years after the first seizure. *Epilepsia* 1978;**19**: 343–50

22. Hertz DG, Ellenberg JH, Nelson KP. The risk of recurrence of nonfebrile seizures in children. *Neurology* 1984;**34**:637–41

23. van den Berg BJ, Yerushally J. Studies on convulsive disorders in young children. *Pediatr Res* 1969;**3**:298–304

6 Management

Medical treatment

The first and most important aspect of treatment is to establish a correct diagnosis of epilepsy and the epilepsy syndrome or seizure type; the second step is to decide that treatment with antiepileptic drugs is necessary; and the third is to decide which drug should be used. The choice of drug depends on the specific epilepsy syndrome or, if no syndrome has been identified, on the type of seizure or seizures experienced by the patient. In the future, the cause of the epilepsy may become the most important factor in helping to determine the choice of drug.

Figure 151 is a diagrammatic representation of the evolution of antiepileptic drugs over time. Most controlled studies have shown no clear benefit of one antiepileptic agent over another; the only obvious exception to this is the proven efficacy of sodium valproate in juvenile myoclonic epilepsy.

Table 6.1 outlines the antiepileptic drugs commonly prescribed in the most frequent types of adult and childhood epilepsy. Table 6.2 lists the antiepileptic agents currently under investigation. The toxicity of these compounds should also be considered, particularly if the drugs are of equal efficacy. Patients and their families should receive counselling regarding:

(1) Aims of treatment;

(2) Prognosis and duration of the expected treatment;

(3) Importance of compliance;

(4) Side-effects.

Ideally, patients / parents should be given a written drug information sheet which provides the following information:

(1) Available preparations of the drug;

(2) Dosing schedule;

(3) Method of administration (particularly important for children);

(4) What to do if a dose is missed or vomited;

(5) Which other drugs (including over-the-counter medicines) can be safely given with the antiepileptic drug(s);

(6) Likely and potential adverse side-effects and what to do if they are experienced.

The initial dose of the chosen drug should be the lowest possible that will achieve seizure control. If necessary, the dose should be increased gradually to the maximum clinically tolerated level

Table 6.1 Most commonly prescribed antiepileptic drugs for the most common types of adult and childhood epilepsy (listed in alphabetical order and not in order of preference)

Epilepsy syndrome or seizure type	Commonly used drug
Idiopathic (primary) generalized, including typical absence, juvenile myoclonic, grand mal on awakening	clobazam/clonazepam* ethosuximide (absences) lamotrigine sodium valproate
Myoclonic–astatic, myoclonic seizures (benign or progressive), and atonic seizures	clobazam/clonazepam ethosuximide lamotrigine sodium valproate
Localization-related[†] (idiopathic/symptomatic), including benign 'rolandic', benign 'occipital' and secondarily generalized	acetazolamide carbamazepine gabapentin lamotrigine phenytoin sodium valproate topiramate vigabatrin
Lennox–Gastaut syndrome[†]	clobazam lamotrigine sodium valproate
Infantile spasms (West's syndrome)[‡]	gammaglobulin (i.v.) nitrazepam prednisolone/ACTH sodium valproate vigabatrin

*The benzodiazepines (clonazepam and nitrazepam more than clobazam) are frequently restricted by tachyphylaxis and tolerance

†Gabapentin has recently become available for adults and is currently under trial in children. Preliminary data with felbamate were encouraging, but the drug is associated with severe (including fatal) aplastic anemia and hepatitis

‡The treatment of infantile spasms is currently under review; ACTH and prednisolone (or betamethasone) are no longer the universally prescribed first drugs. Sodium valproate or nitrazepam are often the first choice in Europe. Vigabatrin has also recently proved effective and is now considered by many (in the UK and Europe) to be the drug of first choice

Table 6.2 New antiepileptic drugs

Drug	Mode of action
Eterobarbital	?increased GABA inhibition
Loreclezole	not known
Losiganone	?enhancement of GABA-mediated inhibition
Oxcarbazepine	limits repetitive firing of sodium-dependent action potentials
Ralitoline	?inactivation of voltage-dependent sodium channel
Remacemide	non-competitive NMDA antagonist
Stiripentol	inhibition of GABA reuptake or metabolism
Tiagabine	inhibition of GABA reuptake
Zonisamide	not known

(irrespective of serum levels) before abandoning its use and transferring the patient to another drug.

Approximately 70% of all patients with epilepsy enter prolonged remission with monotherapy. Comparative studies indicate little difference in efficacy among the commonly used conventional drugs. However, carbamazepine is probably the drug of choice for partial-onset seizures and, despite the absence of controlled data (except in juvenile myoclonic epilepsy), valproate is accepted as the drug of choice for generalized-onset seizures.

There is little evidence of success with dual therapy after failure of optimal doses of a single antiepileptic drug; indeed, seizure control may improve after switching from dual therapy to monotherapy. Furthermore, any improvement in seizure control attributable to the addition of a second drug is likely to be at the expense of increased toxicity.

Complete seizure control with or without evidence of major toxicity is never achieved by 20–25% of

patients. Such patients frequently require a therapeutic compromise (determination of a personalized balance between seizure control and adverse effects). In this group of patients, new antiepileptic drugs or surgery, or both, should be considered.

Meta-analyses of published randomized controlled trials of novel antiepileptic drugs as add-on therapy suggest that lamotrigine and gabapentin are 2.5–3.0 times, vigabatrin and tiagabine 5–6 times, and topiramate 7–8 times more likely than placebo to produce a 50% or greater reduction of seizures. The apparently greater efficacy of topiramate appears to be at the expense of greater toxicity. However, whether or not these findings are genuine or spurious requires direct comparisons between these compounds.

Monitoring the serum levels of antiepileptic drugs is often undertaken, but is only of limited practical use. The therapeutic or target ranges are only guidelines as the optimal level for any given patient may lie well above or below these ranges. In most cases, the dosage of antiepileptic drug is considered appropriate when the patient is seizure-free with no (or at least patient-acceptable) side-effects. Antiepileptic drug levels should be measured in patients who present with status epilepticus, in patients suspected of major non-compliance, or in those receiving polytherapy which includes phenytoin.

Side-effects of antiepileptic drug treatment

Adverse effects with antiepileptic drugs are common. The risk of acute dose-related symptoms and acute idiosyncratic reactions (Table 6.3) can be minimized by cautious dose escalation. Chronic toxicity (Table 6.4) and teratogenicity (Table 6.5) are directly related to high-dose polytherapy.

Some reactions, however, cannot be easily assigned to any of these categories. Incidental mechanisms of action can be important; for example, paresthesia

Table 6.3 Acute anticonvulsant toxicity with antiepileptic drug treatment

Dose-related

Encephalopathy (tiredness, nystagmus, ataxia, dysarthria, confusional state)	phenytoin, carbamazepine, phenobarbitone, benzodiazepines, lamotrigine, gabapentin
Movement disorder	phenytoin
Tremor	valproate

Idiosyncratic

Hypersensitivity	phenytoin, carbamazepine, phenobarbitone, lamotrigine
Aplastic anemia	carbamazepine, phenytoin, felbamate
Acute hepatitis	valproate, phenytoin, phenobarbitone, felbamate
?Acute psychosis	vigabatrin, topiramate

Table 6.4 Chronic anticonvulsant toxicity with antiepileptic drug treatment

Nervous system
Memory and cognitive impairment, hyperactivity and behavior disturbances, pseudodementia, cerebellar atrophy, peripheral neuropathy

Skin
Acne, hirsutism, alopecia, chloasma

Liver
Enzyme induction

Blood
Megaloblastic anemia, thrombocytopenia, pseudolymphoma

Immune system
IgA deficiency, drug-induced systemic lupus erythematosus

Endocrine system
Decreased thyroxine levels, increased cortisol and sex hormone metabolism

Bone
Osteomalacia

Connective tissue
Gingival hypertrophy, coarsened facial features, Dupuytren's contracture

and renal calculi are probably due to the carbonic anhydrase activity of topiramate. Acute psychotic reactions have a multifactorial basis and rarely represent idiosyncratic toxicity.

A non-specific dose-related encephalopathy is common, predictable and reversible. Valproate-induced tremor is common at high doses whereas phenytoin on rare occasions produces a dose-dependent dyskinesia.

Acute idiosyncratic reactions are rare, unpredictable and require immediate drug withdrawal. The risk of hypersensitivity reactions, manifested by rash with or without fever (Figures 152–154), ranges from 2 to 4% whereas Stevens–Johnson syndrome occurs in 1 : 5000–10 000 patients exposed to carbamazepine, phenytoin, phenobarbitone or lamotrigine. Aplastic anemia is an extremely rare complication of phenytoin or carbamazepine ther-

Table 6.5 Teratogenicity of antiepileptic drug treatment

Fetal anticonvulsant syndrome	phenytoin, valproate, trimethadione
Spina bifida	valproate (1–2%), carbamazepine (0.5–1%)

apy whereas acute liver failure attributable to valproate is seen almost exclusively in children < 2 years of age with additional neuropsychiatric handicap. The potent new antiepileptic agent felbamate carries significant risk of fatal hematological or hepatic reactions.

Chronic exposure to antiepileptic drugs can affect any system. A reversible peripheral neuropathy, cerebellar atrophy and osteomalacia are unusual problems essentially confined to institutionalized patients. Cosmetic side-effects attributable to phenytoin or phenobarbitone are particularly troublesome in young women. Gingival hypertrophy is seen in one-third of patients receiving phenytoin (Figure 155).

Women with epilepsy account for 0.5% of all pregnancies. The overall risk of congenital malformations is 4–6%, but is significantly greater in mothers receiving high-dose polytherapy (Figure 156).

A non-specific fetal anticonvulsant syndrome manifested by orofacial clefts, distal digital anomalies (Figure 157) and mild mental handicap with or without cardiac defects has been attributed to several compounds. The risks of neural tube defects with valproate and carbamazepine are 1–2% and 0.5%, respectively.

Although novel drugs are not recommended for pregnant patients, their thorough preclinical evaluation and early clinical data suggest less teratogenicity than with conventional drugs. It must be emphasized, however, that uncontrolled epilepsy presents greater risks than drug therapy to both pregnancy and fetal development.

Holistic management

The management of epilepsy extends far beyond the prescription of antiepileptic medication. For many patients and their families, the social, educational and psychological factors clearly outweigh the issue of seizure control. These needs should be met through a multidisciplinary approach that is preferably carried out within a specialist clinic (for both pediatric and adult patients) with access to education, support and advice from a number of different sources (Table 6.6).

Table 6.6 Multidisciplinary approach to the management of epilepsy

Dedicated and specialist medical staff

Clinical nurse specialist in epilepsy

Clinical psychologist

Psychiatrist

Social worker

Representatives of relevant voluntary associations

Secretarial staff

Status epilepticus

Status epilepticus (SE) can be defined as recurrent epileptic seizures lasting more than 30 min. A practical classification includes the following seizure types:

Tonic-clonic
Absence
Myoclonic
Complex partial (Figures 158 and 159)
Focal motor (epilepsia partialis continua).

Tonic-clonic status epilepticus (TCSE) is a common medical emergency which can be caused by any cerebral pathology, but the causes differ between children and adults (Table 6.7). TCSE produces a characteristic pattern of changes which, ultimately, cause irreversible brain damage and potentially fatal systemic complications. During the first 30 min, compensatory mechanisms ensure that the delivery of glucose to active cerebral tissue is maintained but, when decompensation ensues, worsening systemic hypotension fails to satisfy the demands of cerebral tissue.

The aims of management are cessation of seizures, prevention of complications and treatment/reversal of the underlying cause (Figure 160). The process of management should be in phases which reflect the underlying pathophysiology (Table 6.8).

Table 6.7 Causes of tonic-clonic status epilepticus in children and adults

Children	Adults
Idiopathic (unknown)	non-compliance with
Febrile	anticonvulsants
Acute illness	alcohol
meningitis	drug overdose
encephalitis	stroke
head trauma	metabolic
Abrupt anticonvulsant	tumor
withdrawal	infection
Progressive encephalopathy	unknown

Table 6.8 Management of tonic-clonic status epilepticus (SE)

Stage of SE	Treatment	
	First choice	Alternatives
Early (0–30 min)	lorazepam i.v. / p.r. diazepam i.v. / p.r.	rectal paraldehyde
Established (30–60 min)	phenytoin i.v. phenobarbitone i.v.	?fosphenytoin i.v. chlormethiazole
Refractory (60–90 min)	thiopentone i.v. pentobarbitone i.v.	propofol i.v.

p.r., per rectum, an important alternative route of administration in children when intravenous access is difficult or impossible

In early SE (< 30 min), intravenous benzodiazepine abolishes seizures in 70–80% of cases with a 10–15% rate of hypotension / respiratory depression. Lorazepam is likely to become the drug of first choice because of its rapid onset of action. Rectal paraldehyde may be used in low-dependency settings, such as nursing homes.

In established SE (30–60 min), the patient should be transferred to an emergency treatment unit (ETU). Intravenous phenytoin or phenobarbitone are drugs of choice. Phenobarbitone possesses several advantages, but the prodrug fosphenytoin avoids the tissue-irritant and cardiotoxic effects of phenytoin and, like phenobarbitone, has a rapid onset of action. Chlormethiazole, although effective, is best avoided as its accumulation is associated with a risk of sudden cardiovascular / respiratory collapse.

Patients in refractory SE (60–90 min) require ventilation with full ETU support. The intravenous barbiturates thiopentone and pentobarbitone are the drugs of first choice in these cases. However, although effective, both are associated with unfavorable pharmacokinetics and significant toxicity. The non-barbiturate anesthetic propofol is increasingly being used in ETUs. The relative merits of these different approaches are not yet known but, whichever of these means is adopted, the continuation of usual antiepileptic drug therapy is essential.

Surgical treatment

Surgical intervention is now accepted as a realistic therapeutic option for many patients with medically refractory seizures. Recent advances in presurgical investigation protocols and operative techniques have resulted in a rapid expansion in the number of neuroscience centers performing epilepsy surgery in both Europe and the USA. As a consequence, the number of successfully treated patients continues to rise steadily.

Of the most commonly performed procedures (Table 6.9), the resective procedures are intended to be curative whereas functional operations are essentially palliative. The results of temporal lobe resection are more favorable than extratemporal resection but, in either case, the outcome is dependent on underlying pathology.

Table 6.9 Surgical procedures for refractory seizures

Functional surgery
Stereotactic lesions
   subcortical
   temporal

Disconnection procedures
   corpus callosotomy
   multiple subpial transections

Resective surgery
Temporal lobe resections
   neocorticectomy
   anterior temporal lobectomy
   amygdalohippocampectomy

Extratemporal resections
   frontal
   centroparietal
   occipital

Major resections
   multilobar
   hemispherectomy

Functional procedures

Corpus callosotomy (Figure 161) is the most 'commonly' performed palliative procedure. By disconnecting the epileptogenic cortex from the rest of the brain, damaging secondarily generalized seizures, which are associated with falls, may be abolished in up to 80% of cases although, frequently, the results are far less successful than this. A complex neuropsychological deficit, the disconnection syndrome, can be prevented by anterior resection with sparing of the splenium. The incidence of other sequelae varies, but usually represents exacerbation of preexisting deficits.

Resective procedures

Hemispherectomy This dramatic procedure (Figure 162) is reserved for patients who have a congenital hemiplegia with no useful hand function and refractory seizures or, occasionally, for those with Rasmussen's 'encephalitis'. Complete and sustained remission may be expected in 70–80% of patients. Improvement in contralateral motor function, intellect and behavior may also occur (Figures 163 and 164). A serious delayed complication, cerebral hemosiderosis, occurred in 25–33% of patients after anatomical hemispherectomy, but this problem has been overcome by modified (functional) procedures.

Focal resections The temporal lobe is the most common source of refractory partial seizures. A relatively homogeneous electroclinical temporal lobe 'syndrome' with a specific pathological substrate (Ammon's horn sclerosis) has been identified. This is not the case for extratemporal seizures. Unlike seizures of frontal lobe origin, temporal lobe seizures are easy to lateralize and, unlike the parietal and occipital lobes, the temporal lobe can be removed with relative impunity. Consequently, temporal lobe resections account for approximately two-thirds of all operations performed for intractable epilepsy and are associated with a better postoperative outcome than are extratemporal resections.

Temporal lobe surgery

There are no accurate estimates of the number of patients who might benefit from temporal lobe surgery. However, the available epidemiological data (Table 6.10) suggest that, in the UK, there is a reservoir of approximately 16 000 patients who have a history consistent with Ammon's horn sclerosis and that approximately 1000 new patients per year may present with this condition. In addition, there are likely to be several thousands of patients with definable structural abnormalities, mainly indolent tumors.

Table 6.10 Estimated incidence and prevalence of Ammon's horn sclerosis in the UK

	$n/10^5$ population annually	Case total (n)
Prevalence		
Active epilepsy		400 000
Complex partial seizures		160 000
Drug-resistant CPS		80 000
with history of prolonged early 'febrile' convulsions		16 000
Incidence		
All new cases of epilepsy	50	30 000
Complex partial seizures	20	12 000
Likely to prove refractory	10	6000
with history of prolonged early 'febrile' convulsions	2	1200

CPS, complex partial seizures

Presurgical evaluation

Suitability for temporal lobe resection requires lateralization of seizure onset by imaging and EEG techniques, and exclusion of predictable surgical risks by neuropsychological examination. Although conventional CT scanning can detect gross pathology, this modality has been superseded by MRI, which is superior in detecting small structural and atrophic lesions. Asymmetry of medial temporal structures, demonstrated by MRI-based hippocampal volumetry, is highly correlated with histopathology and postoperative outcome. Postoperative MRI (Figure 165) is a useful method of demonstrating the completeness of resection.

Positron emission tomography (PET) scanning demonstrates hypometabolism in epileptic foci interictally and is a reliable indicator of the site of epileptogenic lesions. However, PET scanners are expensive to install and operate, and ictal events are not easily recorded with this technique. Consequently, this modality is not likely to become generally available. HMPAO–SPECT (hexamethylpropylene amine oxide–single-photon emission computed tomography) scans reveal hypoperfusion in epileptic foci interictally and hyperperfusion postictally. Comparison of interictal and ictal SPECT images (Figure 166) is highly predictive of the seizure focus. In some centers, concordance between interictal EEG, MRI, SPECT and psychometry obviates the need for invasive ictal monitoring. This technique may also be of value in deciding on the placement of depth (intracerebral) electrodes when investigating seizures of extratemporal origin.

Electroencephalography

EEG remains the primary means of preoperative localization. A well-localized interictal anterior temporal spike focus (Figure 167) provides useful localizing information. However, bilateral independent spike foci are common and unilateral foci may be falsely lateralizing. Multicontact foramen ovale electrodes (Figure 168) are now accepted as a useful means for lateralizing seizures with suspected medial temporal onset (Figure 169). Subdural and depth electrodes provide a means of recording from large areas of cortex, and are probably best reserved for differentiating between temporal and extratemporal seizure onsets.

Surgical pathology

Hemispherectomy

The distribution of pathologies for which hemispherectomy is performed is changing with time. Whereas early series were dominated by atrophic lesions secondary to infection or vascular accidents, recent reports reveal that hemimegalencephaly, Sturge–Weber syndrome and Rasmussen's 'encephalitis' are the most common underlying lesions.

Focal resections

There is a broad spectrum of pathological substrates underlying focal epilepsy (Table 6.11). Formerly, extratemporal lesions were almost exclusively post-traumatic or postinfective scars (Figure 170) or tumors with a relatively high proportion of aggressive lesions, whereas temporal lobe resections usually revealed Ammon's horn sclerosis or indolent tumors. More recently, reports reveal an increasing proportion of developmental anomalies, the most common of which is focal cortical dysplasia (Figure 171), most frequently found in frontal and central regions. Vascular malformations (Figures 172 and 173), which can arise at any site, account for a small proportion of cases of temporal lobe epilepsy.

The terminology used to describe the neuropathology of temporal lobe epilepsy has, until recently, been very confusing. However, improved surgical techniques allowing preservation of hippocampal specimens and advances in histopathological diagnosis have contributed to the production of an acceptable classification system (Table 6.12).

Ammon's horn sclerosis. Classical Ammon's horn sclerosis involves varying degrees of neuronal cell loss and gliosis in the CA1 and CA4 regions of the hippocampus and dentate gyrus (Figures 174 and 175). The condition is the cause of approximately 20% of cases of all refractory temporal lobe epilepsy. Ammon's horn sclerosis also accounts for 22–70% of cases in large surgical series. The variability may be due to presurgical selection, but the disorder is consistently the most common entity.

There is strong epidemiological and histopathological evidence to link prolonged early 'febrile' convulsions and Ammon's horn sclerosis. Although some authors contend that the relationship is casual, it is equally likely that the severity of the 'febrile' convulsions and the refractory complex partial seizures

Table 6.11 Structural lesions associated with epilepsy

Malformative
Cortical dysplasia
   microdysgenesis (Meencke)
   focal dysplasia
   cortical dysplasia with hamartomatous proliferation
     of neuroectodermal cells
   polymicrogyria
   lissencephaly / pachygyria
   hemimegalencephaly
Vascular malformations
   arteriovenous
   cavernous hemangioma

Neoplastic
Glioma
Ganglioglioma
Metastatic tumor
Dysembryoplastic neuroepithelial tumor (DNET)
Other

Familial and metabolic
With focal lesions; phakomatosis
   tuberous sclerosis
   neurofibromatosis
   encephalotrigeminal angiomatosis,
     Sturge–Weber syndrome
With diffuse lesions
   lysosomal enzyme deficiencies
   peroxisomal disorders
   mitochondrial enzyme disorders
   unknown etiology, e.g. Alexander's disease,
     lipofuscinosis, myelinopathies
   Lafora's body disease
   miscellaneous myoclonic epilepsies

Cerebrovascular disease and trauma
Ischemic
Hemorrhagic
Post-traumatic

Inflammatory / infectious
Fulminant encephalitis, e.g. due to herpesvirus
Chronic, e.g. parasitic
Rasmussen's 'encephalitis'

Ammon's horn (hippocampal) sclerosis

Table 6.12 Classification of lesions of the temporal lobe in intractable complex partial seizures

(1) Ammon's horn sclerosis
  a. Classical
  b. End folium
(2) Neoplastic lesions
  a. Mixed tumors
    i. Ganglioglioma
    ii. Dysembryoplastic neuroepithelial tumor
    iii. Mixed glial tumors
  b. Gliomas
(3) Familial and metabolic diseases
  a. With focal lesions; phakomatosis
(4) Malformative lesions
  a. Cortical dysplasias
    i. Focal cortical dysplasia
    ii. Microdysgenesis
  b. Vascular malformations
    i. Arteriovenous malformations
    ii. Cavernous malformations
(5) Cerebrovascular disease and trauma
(6) Inflammatory / infectious
  a. Fulminant encephalitis, meningitis
  b. Chronic encephalitis, meningitis
  c. Rasmussen's 'encephalitis'
(7) Non-specific lesions

With permission, from Vinters HV, Armstrong DL, Babb TL, *et al.* The neuropathology of human symptomatic epilepsy. In: Engel J Jr, ed. *Surgical Treatment of the Epilepsies.* New York: Raven Press, 1993

are symptomatic of prenatally acquired cerebral damage. It is also likely that a number of 'febrile' seizures are not temperature-related but are, in fact, unprovoked epileptic seizures.

The CT scan is often normal, but hippocampal atrophy can be readily detected by MRI (Figure 176). The degree of hippocampal asymmetry can be calculated using volumetric studies. Postoperatively,

two-thirds of patients are rendered seizure-free and it has been suggested that diffuse sclerosis, involving the posterior hippocampus, is associated with a poorer outcome.

Neoplastic conditions Indolent tumors are reported in 13–56% of large surgical series. Their increased representation in recent reports probably reflects the wider availability of high-quality MRI. Although these lesions have similar radiological appearances, this category is pathologically heterogeneous, with relatively benign lesions predominating because of their propensity to cause refractory partial seizures. Low-grade gliomas (astrocytoma, oligodendroglioma), mixed cell tumors and anaplastic gliomas account for 60–70%, 20–30% and 10% of cases, respectively.

The mixed cell tumors have a limited growth potential and may not be truly neoplastic. The most common lesion, ganglioglioma (Figures 177 and 178), rarely undergoes malignant transformation. The recently described dysembryoplastic neuroepithelial tumor is becoming increasingly recognized. These lesions typically cause refractory complex partial seizures with onset before age 20 years in neurologically normal individuals who have no evidence of a neurocutaneous syndrome. Their intracortical location is best determined by MRI (Figure 179).

The pathology of these tumors consists of glial nodules, foci of cortical dysplasia and a unique glioneuronal component with a characteristic appearance (Figures 180 and 181). They may resemble both ganglioglioma and true astrocytoma, but distinction from the latter can be made on both clinical and radiological grounds. At least 80% of patients are rendered seizure-free after resection of these lesions.

Focal cortical dysplasia Focal cortical dysplasia is the most common developmental disorder causing epilepsy. Although extratemporal lesions predominate, this pathology is reported in 6–20% of cases of temporal lobe epilepsy. The lesions are highly epileptogenic, causing refractory epilepsy in up to 90% of patients; a history of status epilepticus is obtainable in up to one-third of cases.

MRI (Figure 182) reveals focal areas of cortical thickening, poor gray–white matter differentiation and shallow sulci. A spectrum of pathology has been identified (Figures 183 and 184), ranging from mild cortical disorganization to lesions displaying abnormalities of neuronal migration, cellular division and differentiation. The outcome of surgery depends on the extent of resection, degree of dysplasia and postexcisional EEG appearances. Temporal lobe lesions have a more favorable outcome.

Malformations These are characterized by disorganization of the cytoarchitecture of the brain or its vessels. Microdysgenesis is not visible radiologically, but has recently been described in isolation and in association with other pathology in patients with temporal lobe epilepsy and in patients with generalized epilepsy. Thus, an independent etiological role in focal epilepsy has not been defined. Vascular and arteriovenous malformations, and cavernous angiomas account for 2–10% of cases in reported series. Cavernomas may be familial and multiple.

Miscellaneous Strokes, meningitis and encephalitis rarely cause single focal resectable lesions. Post-traumatic cerebral contusion and focal scarring as a consequence of a cerebral abscess account for a small proportion of surgical cases. Non-specific pathology was formerly reported in 20–30% of large series. These patients consistently had the poorest outcome. However, careful presurgical selection and improved operative techniques have reduced the incidence of negative histology in recent reports.

Dual pathology

With the continuing development of sophisticated neuroimaging modalities (both structural and functional), a number of patients with intractable (predominantly partial) epilepsy have been found to have evidence of dual pathology – hippocampal atrophy or mesial temporal sclerosis **and** another lesion. The most frequently encountered 'other' lesions include a neuronal migration disorder (usually malformations of cortical development or cortical dysplasia) and porencephalic cysts. Less common 'other' lesions include low-grade tumors, vascular malformations and periventricular leukomalacia.

Dual pathology is seen in patients of all ages, including young children (Figure 185). The precise etiology and relationship of the two pathologies are as yet unclear, but it is possible that they share a common pathogenetic mechanism with onset during pre- or perinatal development.

Alternatively, one may have caused the other. The extratemporal lesion (for example, cortical dysplasia) may be responsible for initiating early-onset, frequent, repeated and prolonged seizures (with or without associated febrile illness) which consequently cause, or at least contribute to, the mesial temporal sclerosis.

Dual pathology is clearly an important phenomenon requiring further clarification, as it has significant implications when planning surgical treatment for lesional epilepsy[1,2].

References

1. Cendes F, Cook MJ, Watson C, *et al.* Frequency and characteristics of dual pathology in patients with lesional epilepsy. *Neurology* 1995;**45**: 2058–64.

2. Wyllie E, Comair Y, Ruggieri P, Raja S, Prayson R. Epilepsy surgery in the setting of periventricular leukomalacia and focal cortical dysplasia. *Neurology* 1996;**46**:839–41.

Section 2   Epilepsy Illustrated

List of illustrations

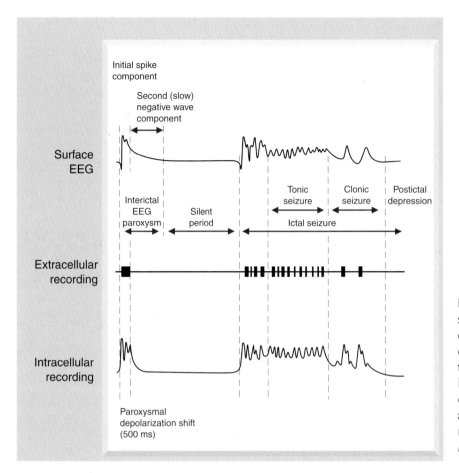

Figure 1 Schematic representation of neurophysiological events in seizure disorders. With permission, from Ayala GF, Matsumoto H, Gumnit RJ. Excitability changes and inhibitory mechanisms in neocortical neurones during seizures. *J Neurophysiol* 1970;33:73–85

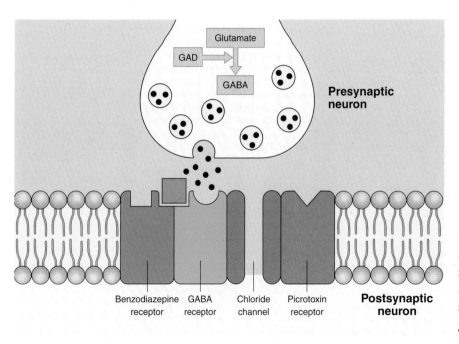

Figure 2 GABA receptor, chloride–ionophore complex and benzodiazepine receptor complex. GABA, gamma-aminobutyric acid; GAD, glutamic acid decarboxylase

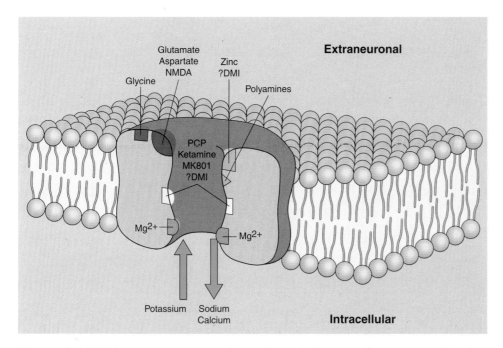

Figure 3 NMDA receptor-operated ion channel showing the variety of binding sites. DMI, desmethylimipramine; PCP, phencyclidine; Zn, zinc; Mg, magnesium

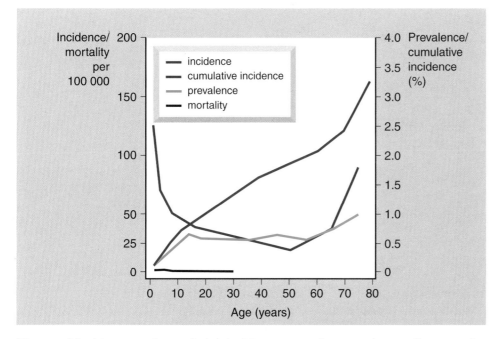

Figure 4 Incidence and cumulative incidence, prevalence and mortality rates for epilepsy in the Rochester, Minnesota (1935–1974) study. With permission from Anderson VE, Hauser WA, Rich S. Genetic heterogeneity of the epilepsies. In: Delgado-Escueta A-V *et al.*, eds. *Advances in Neurology*, vol 44. New York: Raven Press, 1986:59–76

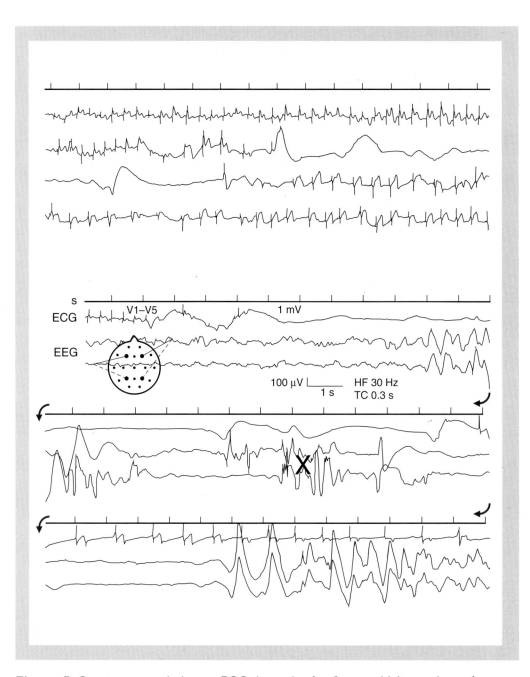

Figure 5 Continuous ambulatory ECG (upper) of a 2-year-old boy, whose frequent episodes of loss of consciousness with rigidity began at age 9 months, taken during a seizure induced by a head bump; such an association with head bumps or other painful stimuli was not recognized for many months. From top to bottom: a time marker (s); consecutive 16-s epochs; 14-s asystole preceded by 3 s of relative bradycardia. The simultaneous EEG (not shown) showed 6–7 s of electrical silence. Cassette EEG/ECG (lower) of a tonic seizure induced by a head bump. Onset of asystole is preceded by 2 s of relative bradycardia and followed by, after 20 s of standstill, a nodal escape rhythm. EEG flattening lasts for 18 s before the abrupt return of cerebral activity 6 s after restoration of ECG. There is no 'epileptic' spiking. With permission, modified from Stephenson JBP. *Fits and Faints*. London: MacKeith Press, 1990:103

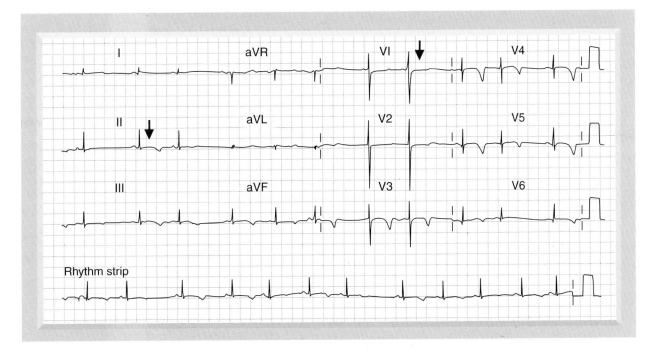

Figure 6 ECG of an 11-year-old boy who had frequent episodes of blackouts or 'faints', particularly during sports and athletics. There is prolongation of the QT interval (arrowed). A similar appearance was seen in his father's ECG. The diagnosis was Romano–Ward syndrome (congenital prolongation of the QT interval)

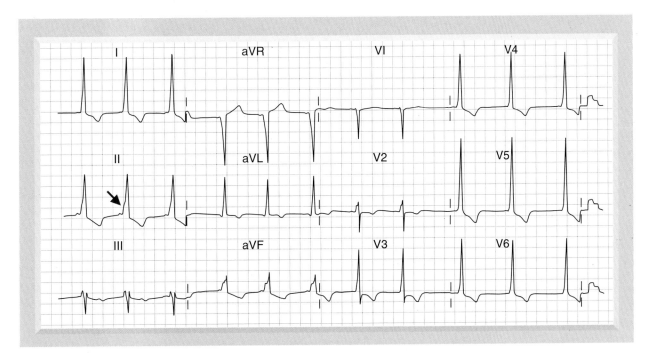

Figure 7 ECG of a 12-year-old boy whose infrequent 'blackouts' were treated as epilepsy with phenytoin. ECG shows Wolff–Parkinson–White syndrome with a short PR interval and delta wave (arrow)

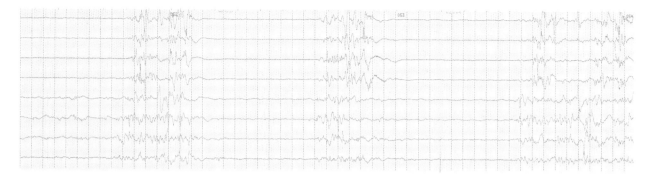

Figure 8 EEG of a 4-week-old girl, whose frequent, daily myoclonic and tonic seizures developed from day 3 of life (early myoclonic encephalopathy) and were resistant to anti-epileptic drugs. This is essentially a burst-suppression pattern, with some of the burst activity accompanied by myoclonias of the head and limbs. (Her CT and metabolic investigations were normal; MRI at age 4 months showed polymicrogyria of both frontal lobes). The patient died at 13 months of age. From top to bottom: Fp2–F4, F4–C4, C4–P4, P4–02; Fp1–F3, F3–C3, C3–P3 and P3–01

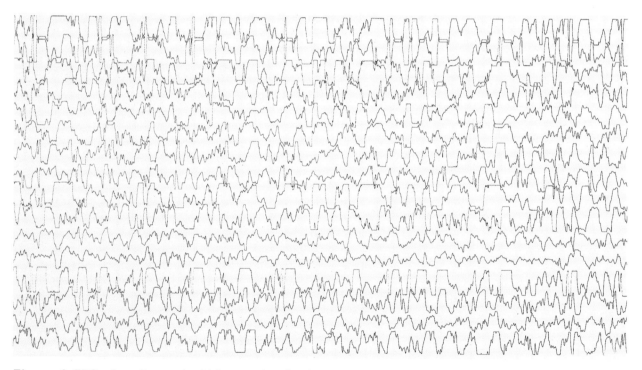

Figure 9 EEG of an 8-month-old boy with infantile spasms and developmental delay (West's syndrome) due to tuberous sclerosis. There is hypsarrhythmia (chaotic disorganized background, multifocal high-amplitude spikes and slow waves). From top to bottom: Fp2–T4, T4–02; Fp1–T3, T3–01; Fp2–F4, F4–C4, C4–P4, P4–02; Fp1–F3, F3–C3, C3–P3, P3–01; T4–C4, C4–Cz, Cz–C3 and C3–T3

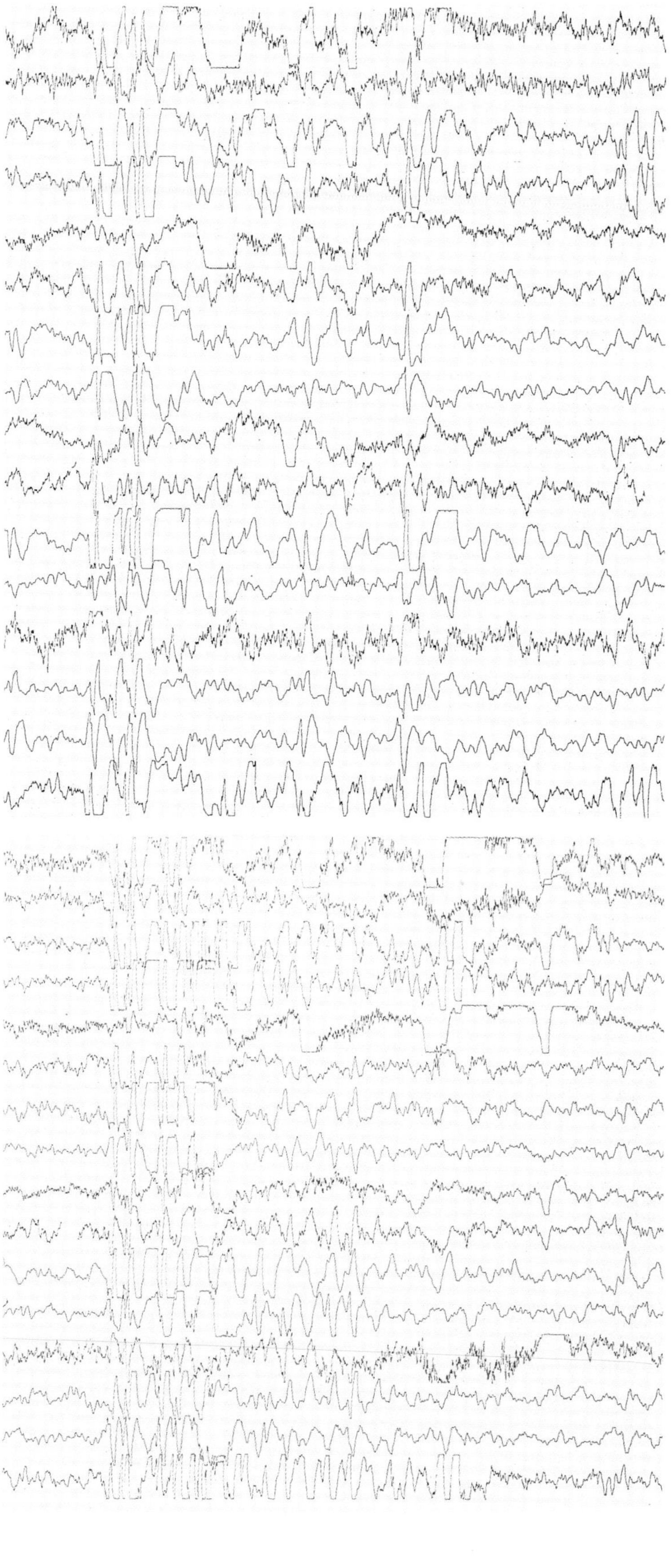

Figure 10 EEGs of a 3-year-old girl with myoclonic-astatic epilepsy showing generalized spike and slow-wave activity, and polyspike discharge accompanied by slight head-drop and knee-jerks (upper); a further similar discharge is accompanied by a jerk backwards with both arms outstretched (lower). From top to bottom: Fp2–T4, T4–02; Fp1–T3, T3–01; Fp2–F4, F4–C4, C4–P4, P4–02; Fp1–F3, F3–C3, C3–P3, P3–01; T4–C4, C4–Cz, Cz–C3 and C3–T3

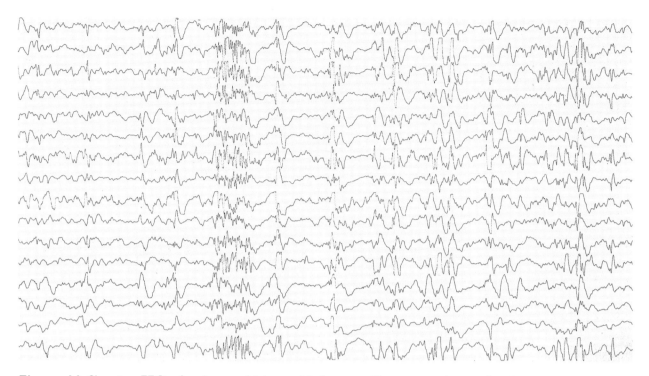

Figure 11 Sleeping EEG of a 6-year-old boy with Lennox–Gastaut syndrome (tonic, atonic, myoclonic and generalized tonic-clonic seizures, and severe learning difficulties) shows multiple discharges of polyspike and spike–wave complexes. From top to bottom: Fp2–F4, F4–C4, C4–P4, P4–02; Fp1–F3, F3–C3, C3–P3, P3–01; Fp2–F8, F8–T4, T4–T6, T6–02; Fp1–F7, F7–T3, T3–T5 and T5–01

Figure 12 EEGs of a 9-year-old boy with Lennox–Gastaut syndrome, who experienced infantile spasms during his first year of life, show irregular diffuse spike and slow-wave activity (lower). This was accompanied by an episode of atypical absence (unresponsive, with twitching of eyelids, chin and fingers) and a burst of rapid rhythm (10 cps) accompanied by a brief 'salaam'-type seizure (upper). From top to bottom: (upper) Fp2–T4, T4–02; Fp1–T3, T3–01; Fp2–F4, F4–C4, C4–P4, P4–02; Fp1–F3, F3–C3, C3–P3, P3–01; T4–C4, C4–Cz, Cz–C3 and C3–T3; (lower) Fp2–T4, T4–02; Fp1–T3, T3–01; Fp2–F4, F4– C4, C4–P4, P4–02; Fp1–F3, F3–C3, C3–P3, P3–01; T4–C4, C4–Cz, Cz–C3 and C3–T3

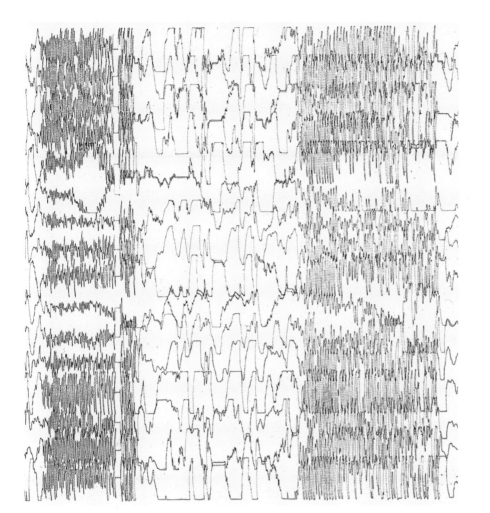

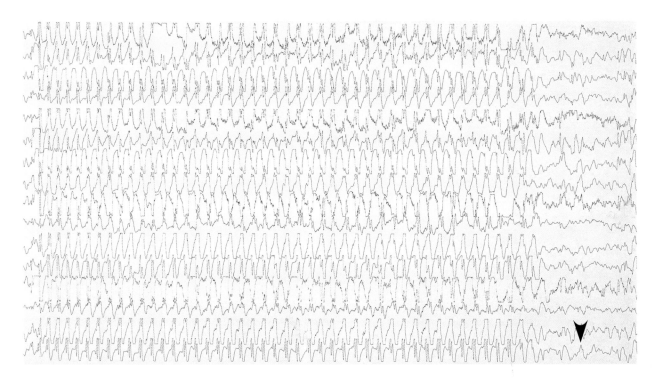

Figure 13 EEG of an 8-year-old girl, who had a 6-week history of 'blanks' and a change in classroom concentration noted by her teacher (childhood-onset typical absence epilepsy), taken during hyperventilation shows generalized spike and slow-wave activity at 3 cps, at which point the patient stopped hyperventilating, opened her eyes and made a couple of lip-smacking movements before resuming hyperventilation 17 s later (arrowed). From top to bottom: Fp2–F4, F4–C4, C4–P4, P4–02; Fp1–F3, F3–C3, C3–P3, P3–01; Fp2–F8, F8–T4, T4–T6, T6–02; Fp1–F7, F7–T3, T3–T5 and T5–01

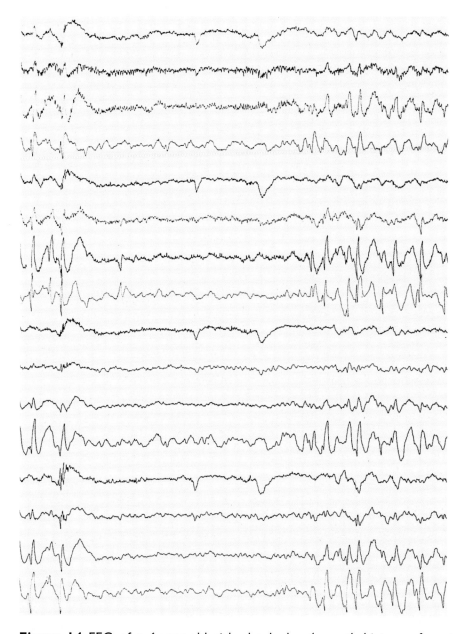

Figure 14 EEG of a 6-year-old girl who had a 4-month history of nocturnal partial seizures characterized by eye deviation, hemiconvulsions and secondary generalization (tonic-clonic convulsions). She also experienced seizures during the day which began with a visual 'aura' (fortification spectra or 'colored lights') and were followed, within 1–2 min, by brief clonic movements (unilateral or bilateral) and a severe headache. Generalized tonic-clonic seizures occasionally followed the initial visual aura. Although migraine was initially diagnosed, the patient in fact has benign childhood epilepsy with occipital paroxysms, comprising high-amplitude runs of repetitive irregular occipital spikes / sharp- and slow-wave complexes occurring bilaterally and tending to attenuate on eye opening (arrowed). From top to bottom: Fp2–F8, F8–T4, T4–T6, T6–02; Fp1–F7, F7–T3, T3–T5, T5–01; Fp2–F4, F4–C4, C4–P4, P4–02; Fp1–F3, F3–C3, C3–P3 and P3–01

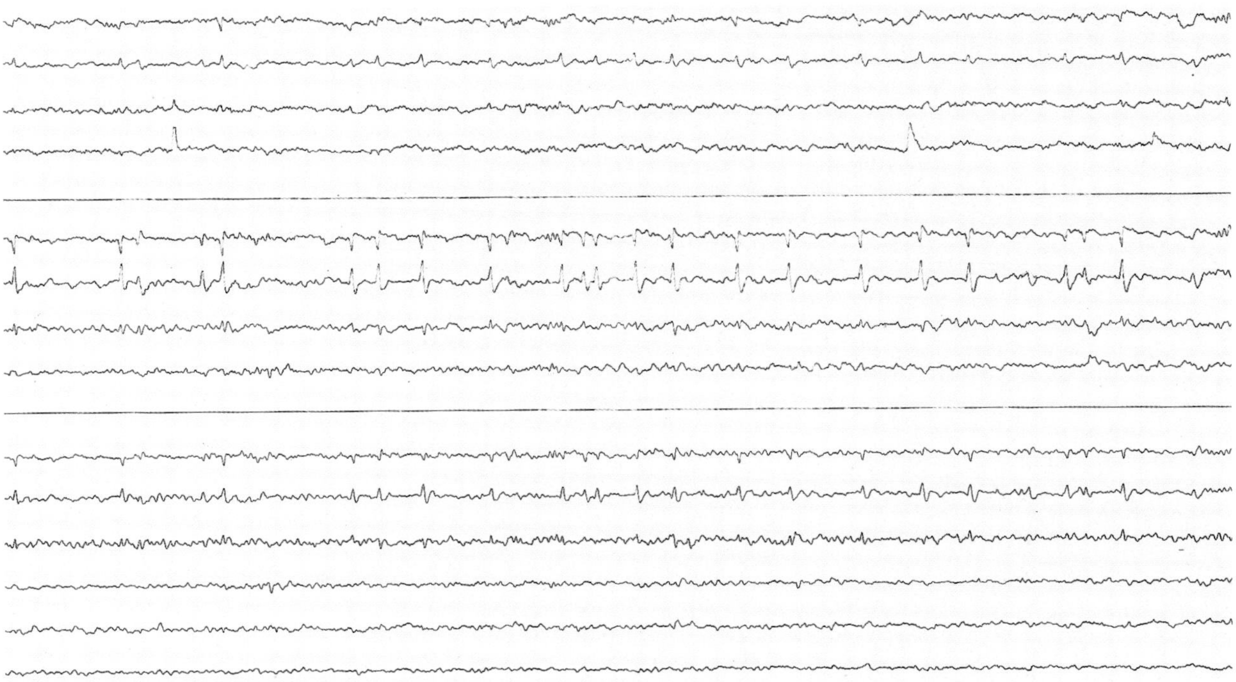

Figure 15 EEG of a 9-year-old boy who had a 6-month history of infrequent partial seizures affecting the tongue, and left side of the face and arm, and one nocturnal generalized tonic-clonic seizure. There is a persistent right centrotemporal sharp-wave discharge (benign partial epilepsy with centrotemporal or rolandic spikes). From top to bottom: F8–F4, F4–Fz, Fz–F3, F3–F7; T4–C4, C4–Cz, Cz–C3, C3–T3; T6–P4, P4–Pz, Pz–P3, P3–T5; Fz–Cz and Cz–Pz

Figure 16 EEGs of a 12-year-old boy with juvenile myoclonic epilepsy showing an irregular spike–wave complex during rest (upper right, facing page), and photosensitivity (unaccompanied by any clinical change) during photic stimulation (lower right, facing page). From top to bottom: Fp2–F4, F4–C4, C4–P4, P4–02; Fp1–F3, F3–C3, C3–P3, P3–01; Fp2–F8, F8–T4, T4–T6, T6–02; Fp1–F7, F7–T3, T3–T5 and T5–01

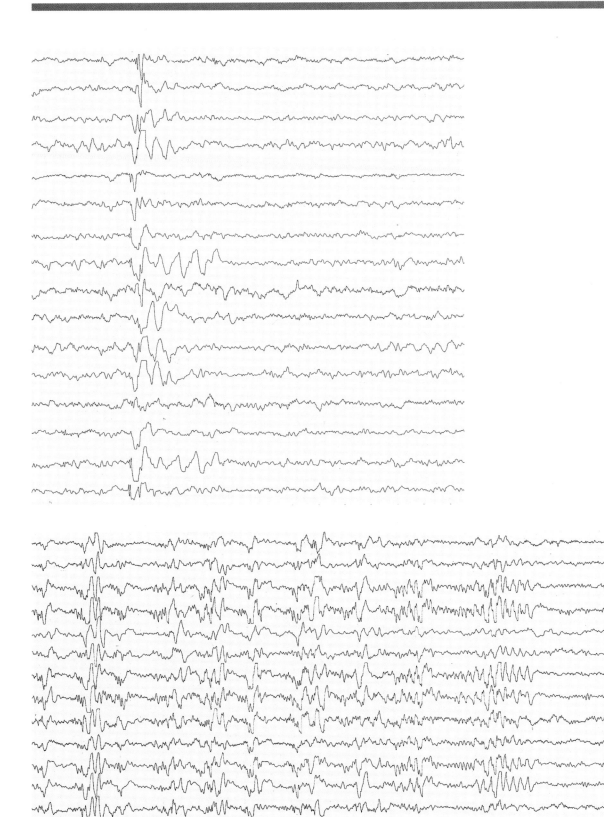

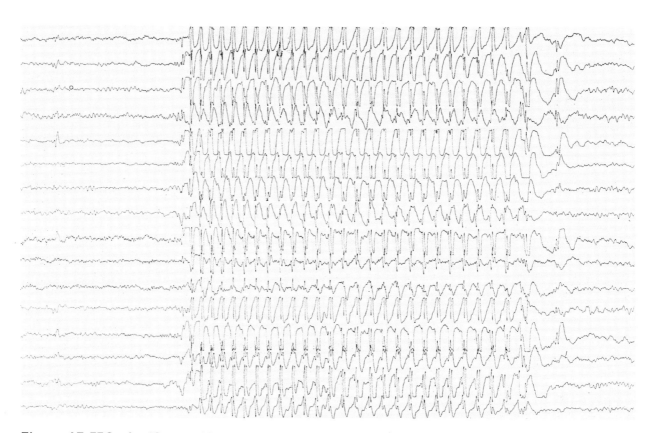

Figure 17 EEG of a 13-year-old girl who had a 6-month history of 'blanks', and two generalized tonic-clonic seizures within a couple of hours of waking (juvenile-onset typical absence epilepsy). There is a generalized discharge of spike and slow-wave activity at 3 cps, accompanied by eye-opening, lip-smacking and a sigh. From top to bottom: Fp2–F4, F4–C4, C4–P4, P4–02; Fp1–F3, F3–C3, C3–P3, P3–01; Fp2–F8, F8–T4, T4–T6, T6–02; Fp1–F7, F7–T3, T3–T5 and T5–01

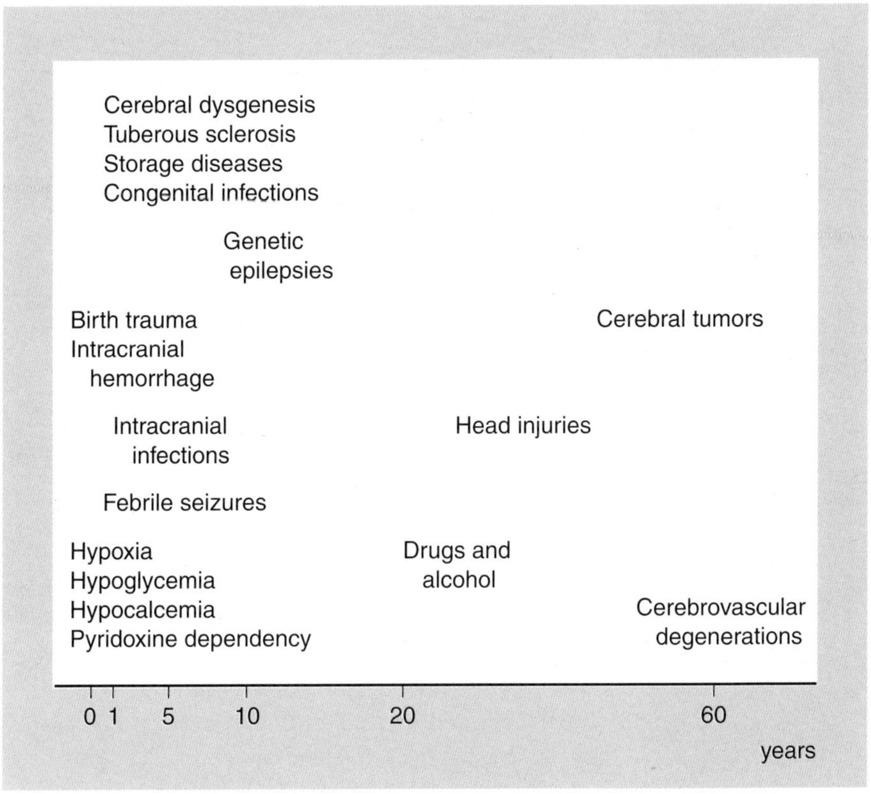

Cerebral dysgenesis
Tuberous sclerosis
Storage diseases
Congenital infections

Genetic
epilepsies

Birth trauma   Cerebral tumors
Intracranial
  hemorrhage

    Intracranial   Head injuries
    infections

  Febrile seizures

Hypoxia   Drugs and
Hypoglycemia   alcohol
Hypocalcemia   Cerebrovascular
Pyridoxine dependency   degenerations

```
0  1    5    10        20                      60
                                            years
```

Figure 18 Causes of seizures and epilepsy by age. With permission, modified from Chadwick D, Cartlidge N, Bates D, eds. *Medical Neurology*. Edinburgh: Churchill Livingstone, 1989

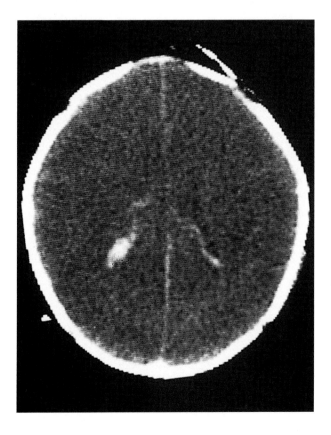

Figure 19 Axial CT of hypoxic–ischemic encephalopathy in a 24-h-old infant, born at week 42 of gestation following an antepartum hemorrhage. The brain is markedly swollen with no white–gray matter differentiation. Seizures developed 4 h after birth and persisted until death 3 days later

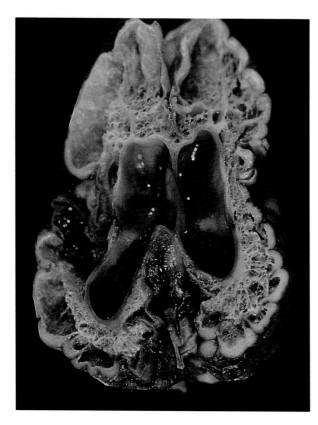

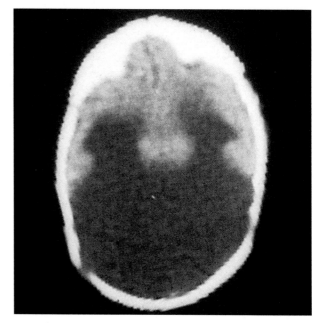

Figure 21 CT of porencephaly shows loss of much of the substance of the cerebrum, which has been replaced by bilateral cystic cavities covered by leptomeninges which communicate with the ventricular system

Figure 20 Cystic encephalomalacia. All of the cerebral white matter has been reduced to a honeycomb of cystic cavities traversed by gliovascular strands

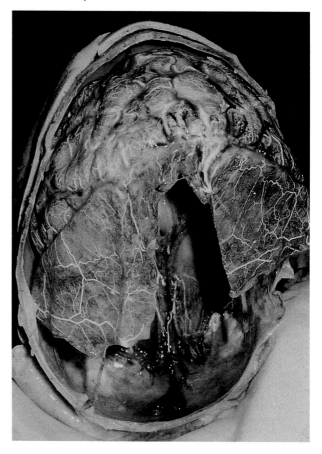

Figure 22 Gross appearance of the cerebrum in porencephaly removed at autopsy

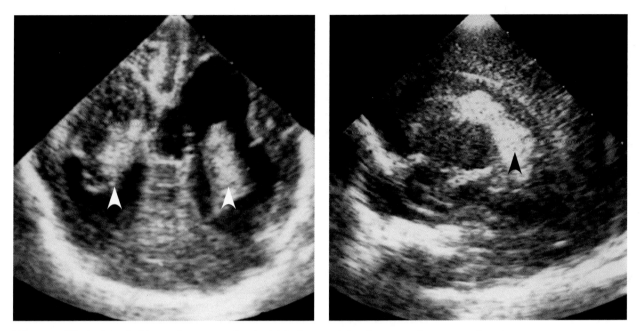

Figure 23 Axial (left) and parasagittal (right) cranial ultrasound scans showing ventricular dilatation and bilateral (left) intraventricular hemorrhages (arrowed) in a 6-day-old infant, born at week 28 of gestation, who presented with seizures, hypotension and sudden collapse

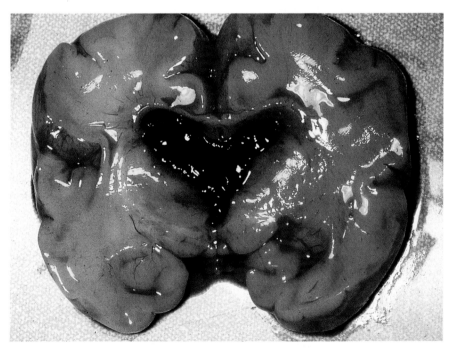

Figure 24 Perinatal intraventricular hemorrhage. A coronal section of brain at the level of the mammillary bodies shows the ventricles to be filled with blood. Hemorrhage into the periventricular germinal matrix and ventricles is common in perinatal hypoxic–ischemic encephalopathies

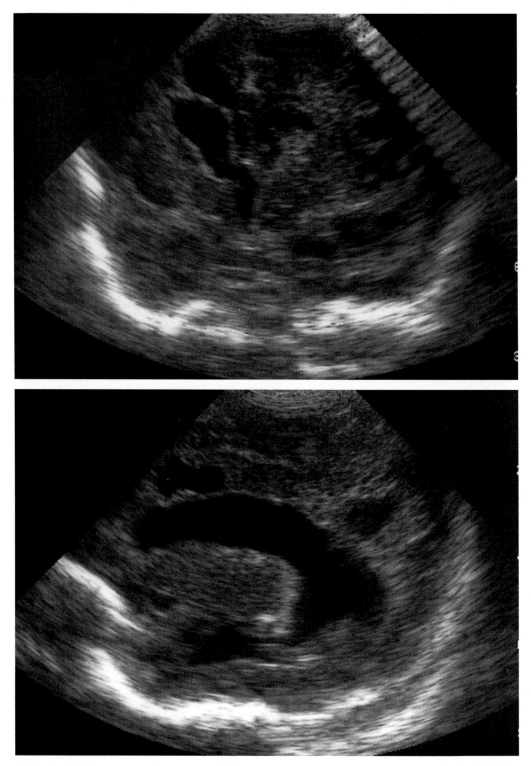

Figure 25 Periventricular leukomalacia. A 3-week-old boy born at week 32 of gestation presented with hypotonia, and frequent tonic and myoclonic seizures due to periventricular leukomalacia following a periventricular hemorrhage. Coronal (upper) and parasagittal (lower) cranial ultrasound scans show irregular and enlarged lateral ventricles and numerous cystic spaces

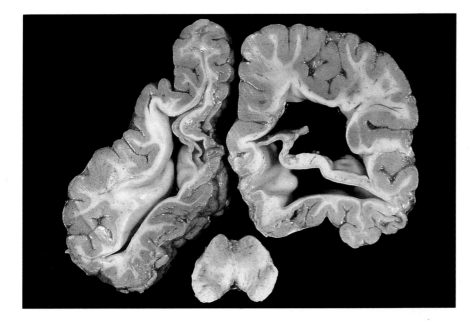

Figure 26 Periventricular leukomalacia. Gross appearance of the cerebrum shows that the damage principally affects the white matter adjacent to the ventricles, resulting in periventricular cavities

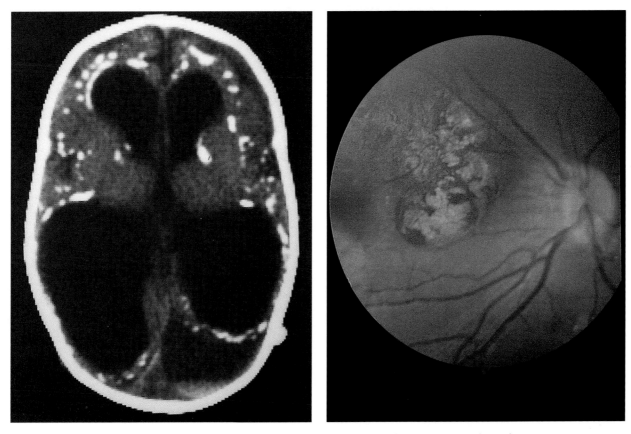

Figure 27 Congenital *Toxoplasma* infection. A 10-month-old boy presented with epilepsy, cortical visual impairment and developmental delay due to congenital *Toxoplasma* infection. Axial CT (left) shows ventriculomegaly (hydrocephalus) and diffuse periventricular calcification; funduscopy (right) reveals gross pigmented chorioretinitis

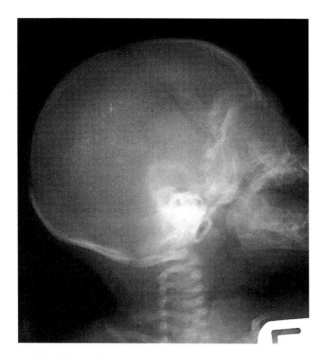

Figure 28 Congenital *Toxoplasma* infection. A 2-day-old infant presented with microcephaly, retinal scarring and repeated tonic seizures. A lateral skull X-ray shows microcephaly and subtle diffuse punctate calcification

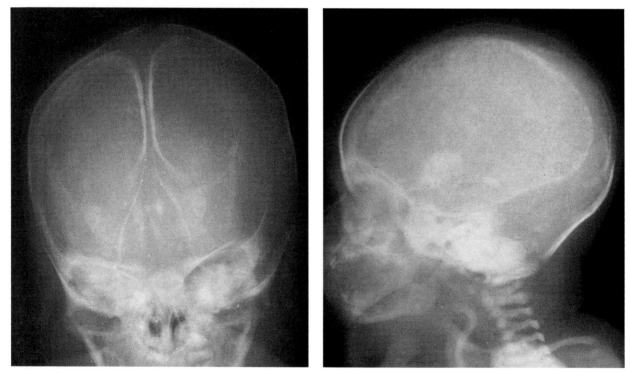

Figure 29 Congenital cytomegalovirus (CMV) infection. A 4-day-old girl presented with microcephaly, retinal scarring (see Figure 30), and frequent tonic and myoclonic seizures due to congenital CMV infection. Anteroposterior (left) and lateral (right) X-rays of the skull show ventriculomegaly and marked, almost continuous, periventricular calcification

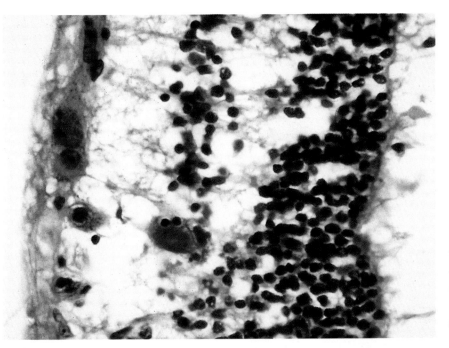

Figure 30 Cytomegalovirus (CMV) retinitis. Histology of the retina shows ganglion cells to contain large intranuclear and smaller granular intracytoplasmic CMV inclusion bodies. (H & E)

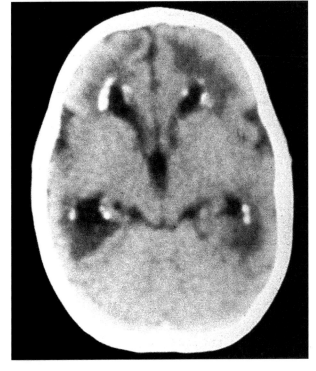

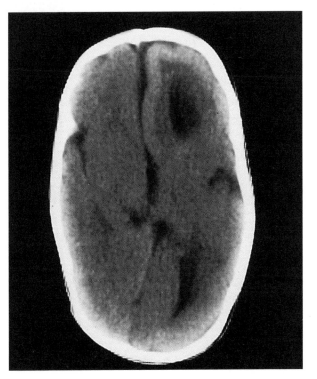

Figure 31 Congenital cytomegalovirus (CMV) infection. A 3-month-old infant presented with microcephaly, and myoclonic and tonic seizures due to congenital CMV infection. Axial non-contrast CT shows periventricular calcification and probable major neuronal migration abnormalities (pachygyria)

Figure 32 Hemimegalencephaly. A 3-week-old infant boy, who presented with drug-resistant intractable seizures, was 'cured' by a left hemispherectomy. Axial CT shows left hemimegalencephaly, and left frontal cortical thickening with pachygyria, prominence of the cortical sulci and dilatation of the left lateral ventricle

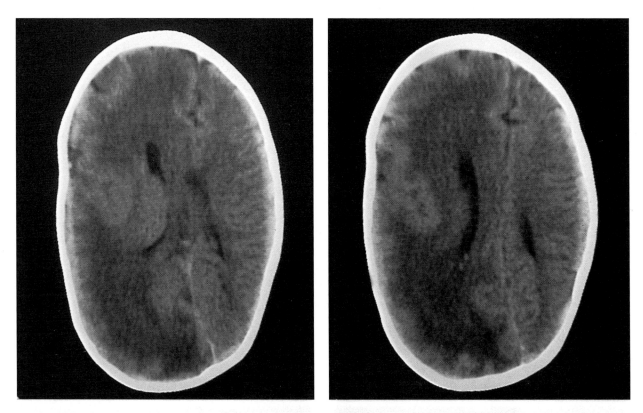

Figure 33 Hemimegalencephaly. A 2½-year-old boy presented with a left hemiparesis, and intractable partial and secondarily generalized seizures. Axial CTs show marked left hemimegalencephaly, with a complete absence of normal myelination and heterotopic islands of gray matter

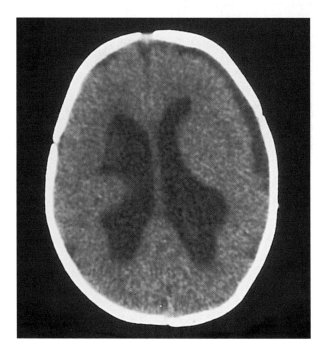

Figure 34 Lissencephaly. A 2-month-old boy presented with microcephaly, an evolving spastic quadriplegia, cortical visual impairment, and daily tonic, clonic and myoclonic seizures. Axial CT shows enlarged dysmorphic ventricles, lissencephaly ('smooth brain') and a coincidental right frontal subdural cerebrospinal fluid collection

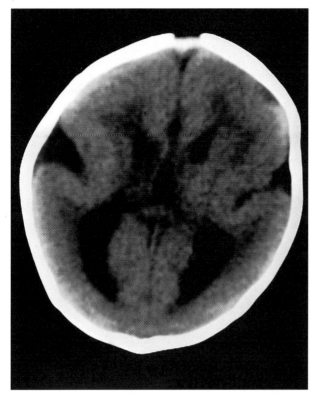

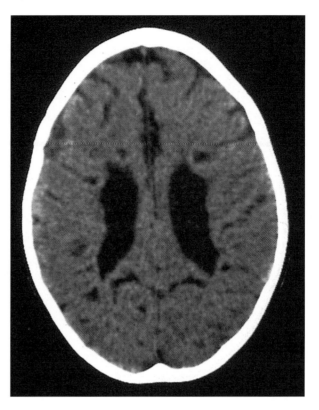

Figure 35 Type I lissencephaly. A 6-week-old boy presented with microcephaly and frequent seizures from birth. Axial CT shows a smooth cortex with an interface between gray and white matter, a thick cortical mantle and a lack of an operculum with open sylvian fissures

Figure 36 Neuronal migration disorder. A 3½-year-old girl presented with persistent seizures, and repeated episodes of convulsive and non-convulsive status epilepticus from age 1 week. Axial CT shows irregular dysmorphic lateral ventricles (probably due to heterotopic gray matter), deep sulci and no discernible white–gray matter differentiation

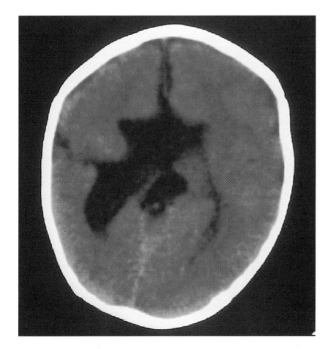

Figure 37 Schizencephaly. A 6-month-old boy presented with developmental delay, cortical visual impairment and infantile spasms. Axial CT shows a major cerebral malformation with unilateral schizencephaly, agenesis of the corpus callosum and an abnormal white–gray matter differentiation, particularly within the left frontal lobe

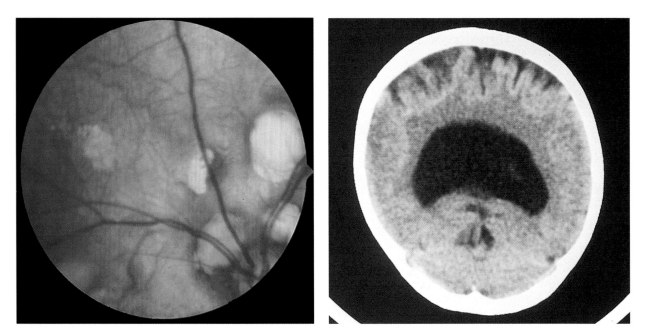

Figure 38 Aicardi syndrome. A 2-year-old girl presented with infantile spasms, frequent partial seizures, profound learning difficulties, cerebral dysgenesis, vertebral abnormalities and chorioretinopathy. Funduscopy (left) shows numerous 'punched-out', hypopigmented retinal lacunae, characteristic of Aicardi syndrome chorioretinopathy. Axial CT (right; same patient) shows semilobar holoprosencephaly, a well-recognized malformation of the syndrome. Both lobar (see **Figure 39**) and alobar (see **Figure 40**) holoprosencephaly may occur. However, the most commonly found malformation in Aicardi syndrome is agenesis of the corpus callosum (see **Figures 41** and **42**)

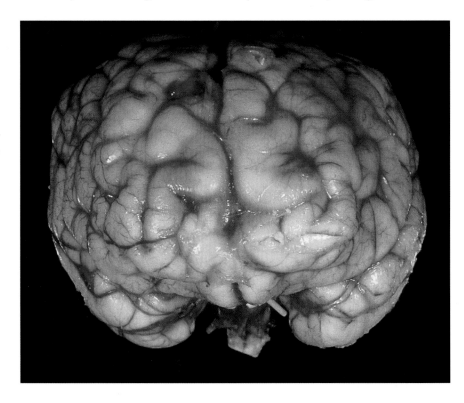

Figure 39 Holoprosencephaly (lobar). Gross appearance of the cerebrum from the front shows an incomplete interhemispheric fissure with fusion of the frontal lobes. Absence of the olfactory bulbs and tracts is apparent

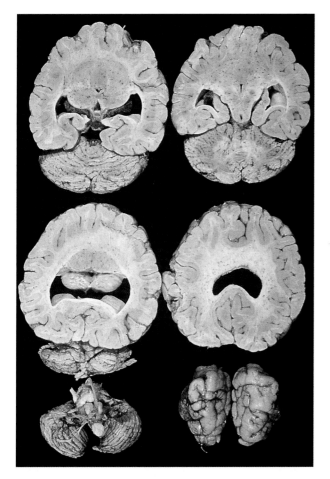

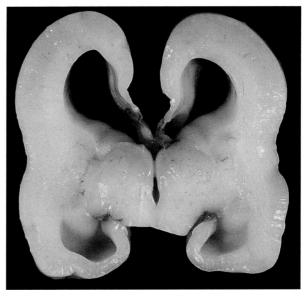

Figure 41 Agenesis of the corpus callosum in a fetus (at approximately week 16 of gestation). The corpus callosum is completely absent. The ventricles are dilated and the hippocampi are poorly formed

Figure 40 Holoprosencephaly (alobar). Multiple coronal sections of the brain reveal only a rudimentary interhemispheric fissure, a large single ventricle and fusion of the deep gray nuclei

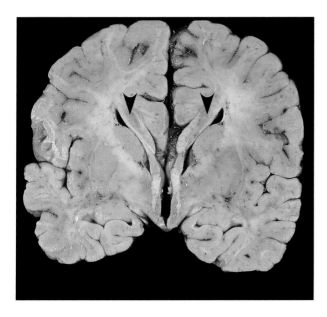

Figure 42 Agenesis of the corpus callosum in a child. The agenesis is complete, and Probst bundles are conspicuous (arrowed)

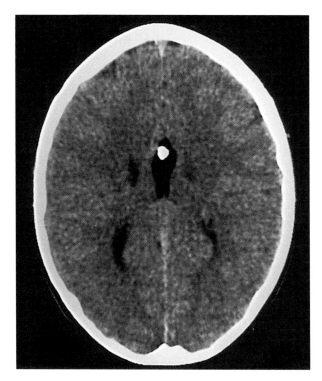

Figure 43 Lipoma of the corpus callosum. A 12-year-old boy presented with infrequent atypical absences. Axial CT shows a midline black area, representing fat, which is denser than the cerebrospinal fluid in the occipital horns of the lateral ventricles. The white lesion is calcification. (Lipoma of the corpus callosum is frequently an incidental finding; the epilepsy in this case may be unrelated to the lipoma)

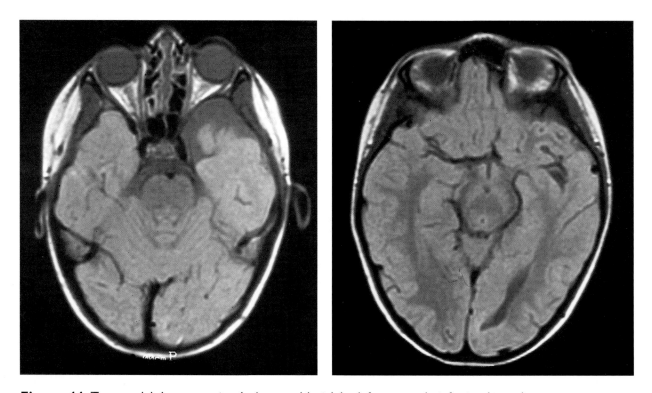

Figure 44 Temporal lobe agenesis. A 6-year-old girl had frequent, brief, simple and complex partial seizures that were controlled by antiepileptic drugs. MRI scans show partial agenesis of the left temporal lobe (left), and dysgenesis of the left temporal and occipital lobes (right)

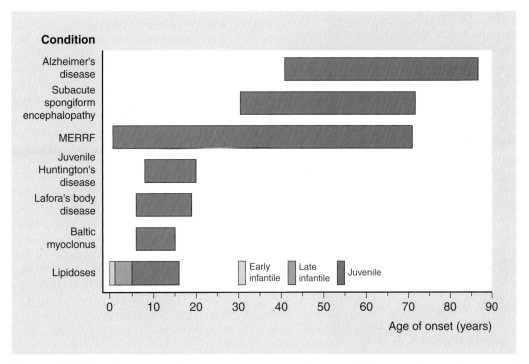

Figure 45 Age of onset of rare neurodegenerative conditions causing seizures and epilepsy

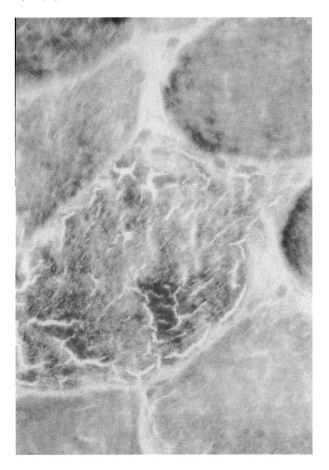

Figure 46 'Ragged red' fibers. A 27-year-old man developed a progressive illness comprising ataxia, myoclonic epilepsy and dementia, which culminated in death after 5 years. Histology of the central fiber in a frozen muscle section shows coarse red staining, indicative of abnormalities of mitochondrial distribution, structure and function. (Gomori trichrome)

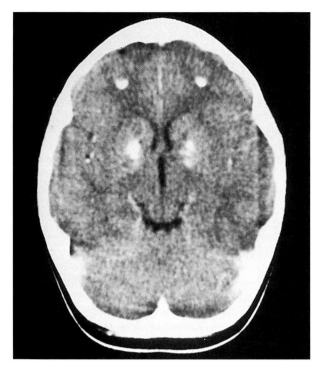

Figure 47 Myoclonic epilepsy with ragged red fibers (MERRF). A 14-year-old boy presented with short stature, learning difficulties and epilepsy (myoclonic and generalized tonic-clonic seizures). Non-contrast axial CT shows symmetrical areas of calcification within the basal ganglia and frontal lobes. (Serum and cerebrospinal fluid showed high levels of lactate, and muscle biopsy revealed ragged red fibers)

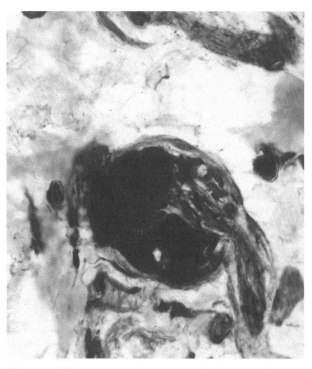

Figure 48 Lysosomal enzyme deficiency. Frozen histological section of rectal biopsy shows the cytoplasm of ganglion cells in the myenteric plexus to be distended by strongly PAS-positive glycolipid. (Periodic acid–Schiff)

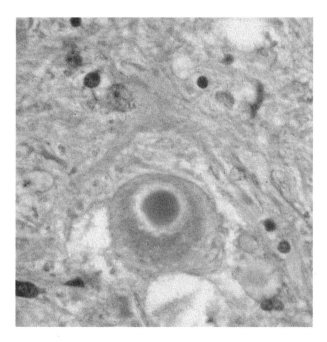

Figure 49 Lafora's body disease. A postmortem was carried out on a teenage gypsy girl with an undiagnosed progressive neurological disorder. She had never been investigated by a neurologist and was found dead in her caravan. This neuron, from the dorsal horn of the spinal cord, contains a large Lafora body in the perikaryon showing the typical central dense zone and lucent halo. The bodies consist of polyglucosan material. (H & E–luxol-fast blue)

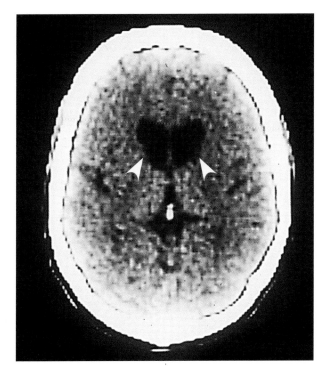

Figure 50 Huntington's disease. A 51-year-old woman presented with dementia, myoclonus and 'restlessness'. Non-contrast axial CT shows the loss of the normal bulge in the inferolateral border of the frontal horn of the lateral ventricle (arrowed). There is also diffuse enlargement of the lateral ventricles

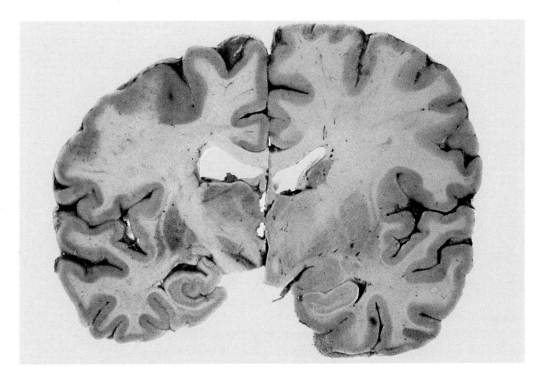

Figure 51 Huntington's disease. Coronal sections taken at the level of the pes hippocampi of a normal cerebrum (right side) and a cerebrum showing the pathological changes of Huntington's disease (left side), namely, near-complete atrophy of the caudate nucleus and, to a lesser extent, of the lentiform nucleus, particularly the putamen

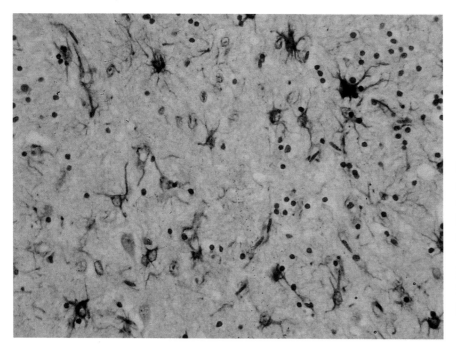

Figure 52 Huntington's disease. Histology of the caudate nucleus shows marked loss of small- and medium-sized neurons, and proliferation of large reactive GFAP-positive astrocytes. [Immunoperoxidase method for glial fibrillary acidic protein (GFAP)]

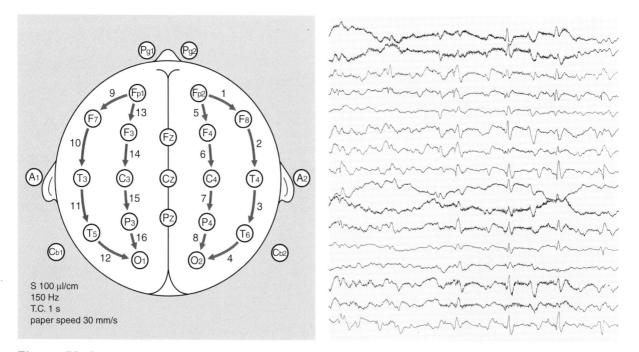

Figure 53 Subacute spongiform encephalopathy. A 62-year-old woman, first seen by a neurologist in a psychiatric unit, initially presented with paranoid ideation, followed by a rapid progressive decline in cognitive function. Examination revealed ataxia, quadriparesis, cortical blindness and multifocal myoclonus. Her EEGs show a diffuse background slow-wave abnormality with relative impoverishment over the left hemisphere and frequent generalized periodic complexes. From top to bottom: Fp2–F8, F8–T4, T4–T6, T6–02; Fp2–F4, F4–C4, C4–P4, P4–02; Fp1–F7, F7–T3, T3–T5, T5–01; Fp1–F3, F3–C3, C3–P3 and P3–01

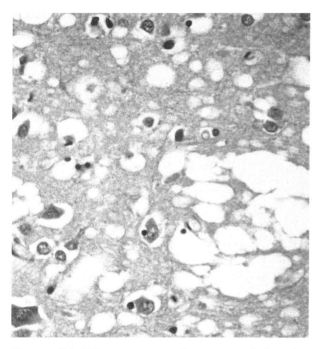

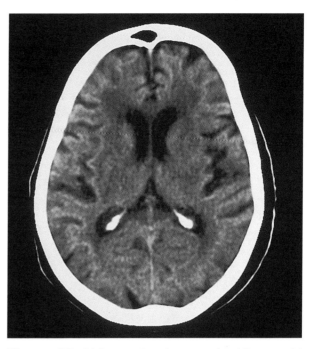

Figure 54 Subacute spongiform encephalopathy. Histology of the cerebral cortex shows the characteristic spongiform change affecting the neuropil between and adjacent to neurons. Two areas of confluent spongy change are particularly conspicuous in this section. In the later stages of the disease, neuronal loss and gliosis can readily be appreciated (not seen here; H & E)

Figure 55 Alzheimer's disease. A 65-year-old woman was brought to a neurology outpatients department by her family, who reported a gradual deterioration of memory over the previous 2 years. Examination revealed disorientation in time and place, and a marked expressive dysphasia. Her CT reveals generalized cerebral atrophy with marked widening of the cortical sulci

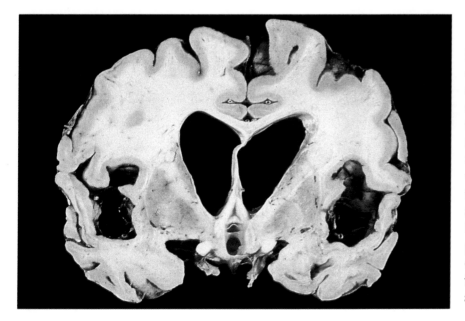

Figure 56 Alzheimer's disease. Coronal section of the cerebrum at the level of the mammillary bodies shows severe cerebral atrophy, most noticeably in the superior temporal gyri, with widening of the fissures, particularly the sylvian fissures, and marked dilatation of the lateral and third ventricles. In patients with Alzheimer's disease, the brain rarely manifests such a severe degree of atrophy at the time of death

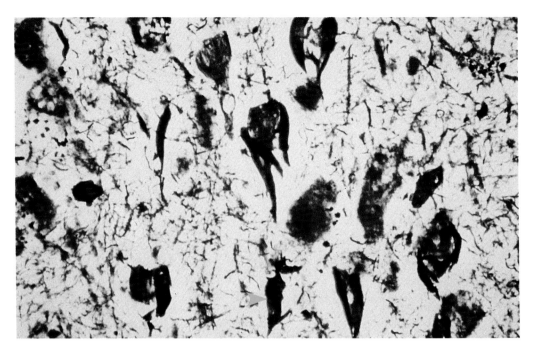

Figure 57 Alzheimer's disease. Histology of the hippocampus shows neurofibrillary tangles (arrowed) in virtually every large neuron. (von Braunmuhl's silver-impregnation technique)

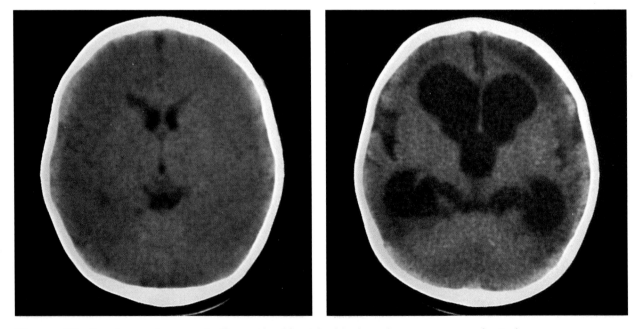

Figure 58 Reye's syndrome. A 7-month-old girl developed severe neurological impairment and intractable epilepsy following Reye's syndrome. Axial CTs show obliteration of normal white–gray matter differentiation (diffuse low-density pattern) at presentation (left), and obstructive hydrocephalus (normal fourth ventricle) with periventricular edema 3 months later (right)

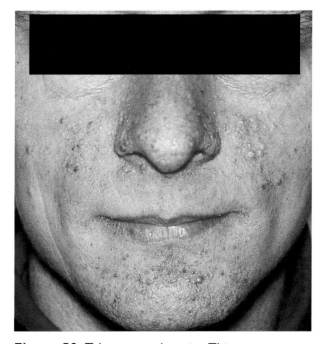

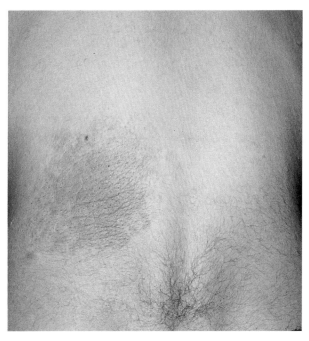

Figure 59 Tuberous sclerosis. This young man with tuberous sclerosis had well-controlled complex partial seizures. Multiple angiofibromas (adenoma sebaceum) are especially prominent in the nasolabial folds

Figure 60 Tuberous sclerosis. The lower back (same patient as in **Figure 59**) reveals a large shagreen patch

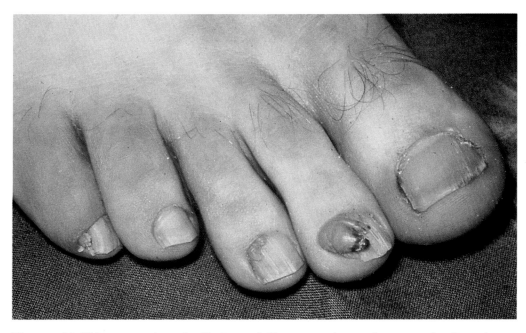

Figure 61 Tuberous sclerosis. Periungual fibromas, shown here on the foot (same patient as in **Figures 59** and **60**) may be the only cutaneous manifestation of tuberous sclerosis. Thus, the feet should always be examined if this diagnosis is suspected

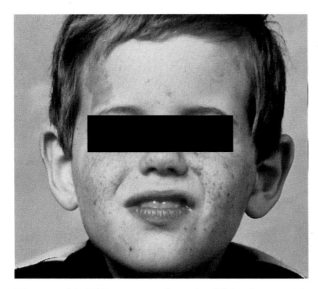

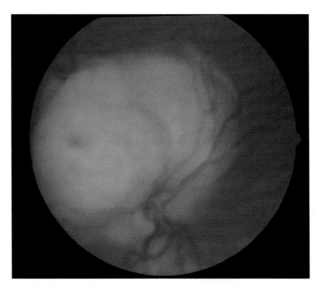

Figure 62 Tuberous sclerosis. This boy with tuberous sclerosis has myoclonic and partial seizures. Angiofibromas (adenoma sebaceum) and a fibrous plaque are seen on the forehead

Figure 63 Tuberous sclerosis. Funduscopy shows a large pale retinal tumor

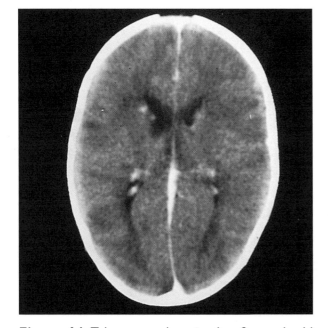

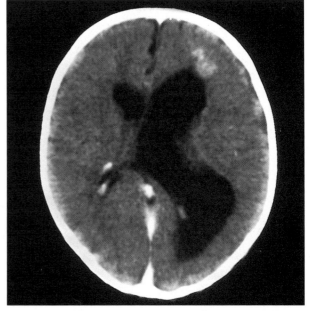

Figure 64 Tuberous sclerosis. An 8-month-old boy presented with infantile spasms and hypsarrhythmia on EEG (West's syndrome) due to tuberous sclerosis. Contrast-enhanced axial CT shows small, but numerous, periventricular calcified tubers or plaques. Multiple low-density phakomas are also present

Figure 65 Tuberous sclerosis. A 9-month-old boy presented with infantile spasms, hypsarrhythmia (on EEG) and developmental delay (West's syndrome) due to tuberous sclerosis. Contrast-enhanced axial CT shows marked asymmetrical ventricular dilatation, and calcified tubers lateral to the frontal horn of the right lateral ventricle and lateral to the occipital horn of the left lateral ventricle

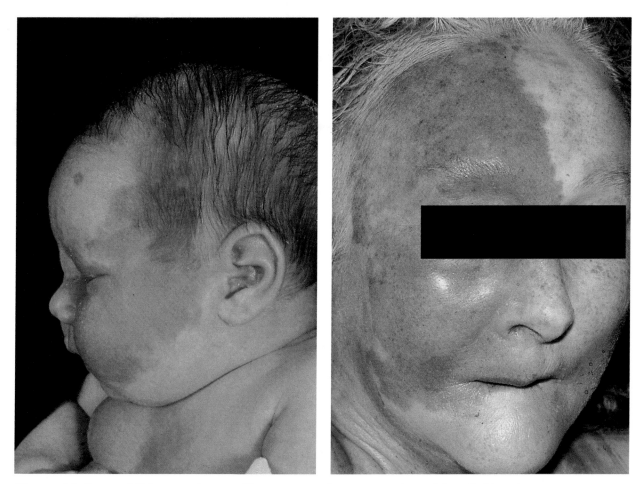

Figure 66 Sturge–Weber syndrome. Cutaneous angiomata seen in an infant (left) and in an adult (right)

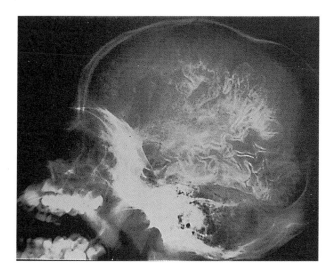

Figure 67 Sturge–Weber syndrome. In an 8-year-old girl with persistent partial seizures due to this neurocutaneous syndrome, a plain lateral skull X-ray shows diffuse, mainly parieto-occipital 'railroad track' or 'tramline' calcification, characteristic of the venous malformation in this syndrome

97

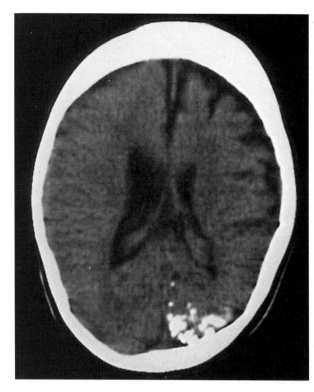

Figure 68 Sturge–Weber syndrome. This 15-year-old girl has an extensive facial nevus with intra-esophageal extension, left hemiparesis, intractable epilepsy and moderate mental handicap. CT shows right hemisphere atrophy with occipital calcification. A year after right hemispherectomy, the patient was seizure-free with significant improvements in both behavior and cognition

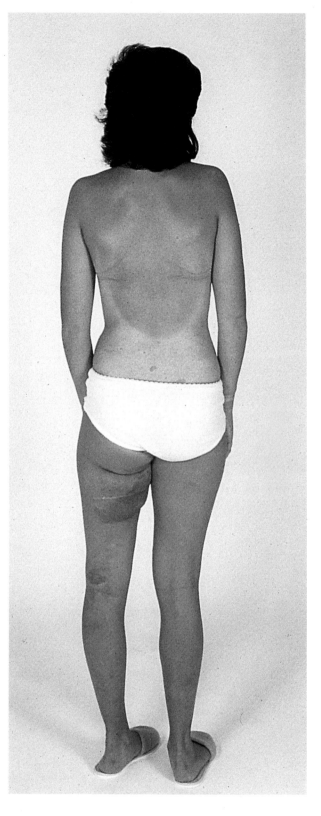

Figure 69 Neurofibromatosis. Café-au-lait spots are present on the trunk and neurofibromata can be seen on the posterior aspect of the left leg

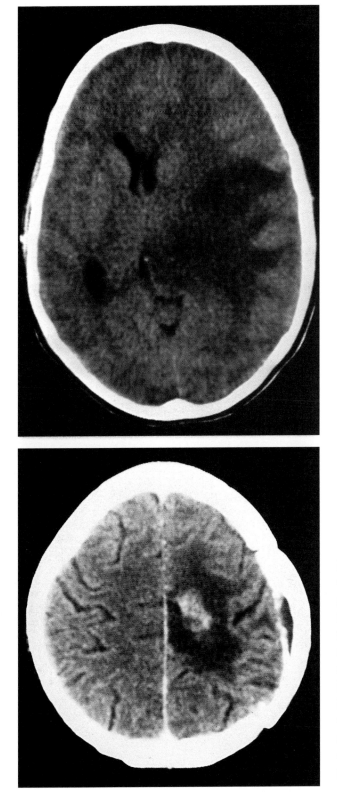

Figure 70 Neurofibromatosis. A 12-year-old girl with type I neurofibromatosis presented with a progressive mild right hemiparesis and two right-sided focal motor-onset, secondarily generalized, seizures. Non-contrast axial CT (upper) shows marked edema of the left hemisphere with midline shift, and compression of the frontal and occipital horns of the left lateral ventricle. CT at a higher level, with contrast (lower), reveals an irregular but well-defined mass within the area of edema. An astrocytoma (grade 1) was completely removed at operation. The patient experienced no further seizures at follow-up 2 years later

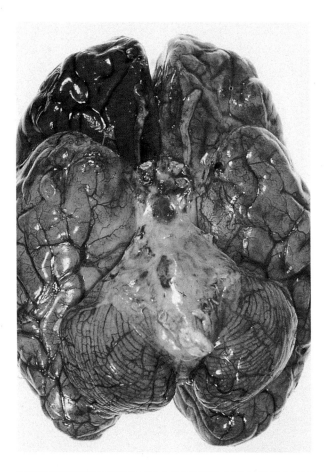

Figure 71 Bacterial meningitis. A 65-year-old male alcoholic was found unconscious in a park. Cerebrospinal fluid examination was consistent with pneumococcal meningitis. Despite appropriate therapy, he succumbed within 48 h. The post-mortem examination confirmed acute bacterial leptomeningitis. The base of the brain shows copious amounts of pus in the subarachnoid space over the brain stem and cerebellum, and in the interpeduncular fossa. The right frontal lobe shows early hemorrhagic infarction

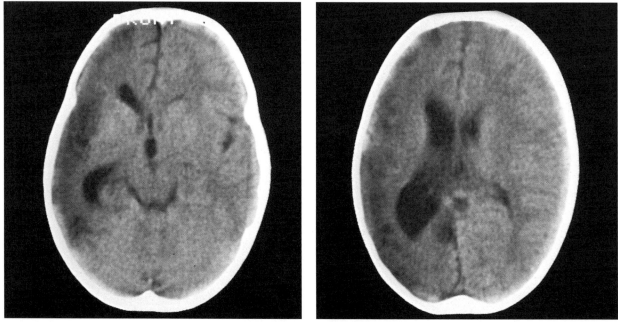

Figure 72 Bacterial meningitis. In a 4¹/₂-year-old girl with right hemiparesis, and partial and secondarily generalized seizures following meningococcal meningitis, axial CTs show infarction of the left hemisphere with consequent 'atrophy' and ventricular enlargement

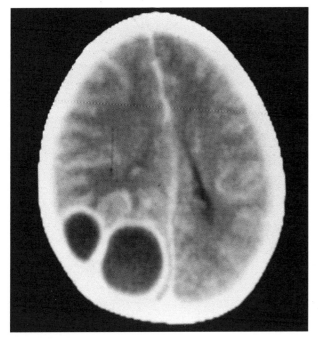

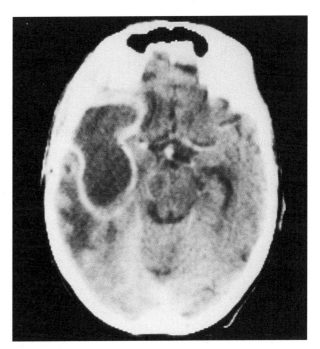

Figure 73 Cerebral abscess. A 4-year-old boy with congenital cyanotic heart disease presented with focal seizures and fever. Contrast-enhanced axial CT shows two well-defined ring-enhancing cerebral abscesses within the left occipital lobe, and some mass effect

Figure 74 Cerebral abscess. Contrast-enhanced CT shows a large biloculated lesion with an enhancing rim and a lower-density center in the right temporal region with surrounding and more posterior edema

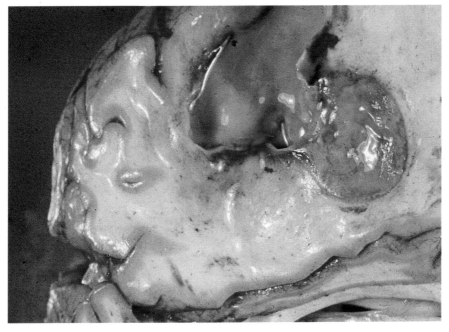

Figure 75 Cerebral abscess. Horizontal section through the right frontal lobe shows a large convoluted abscess with a thick fibrous wall containing an abundance of pus

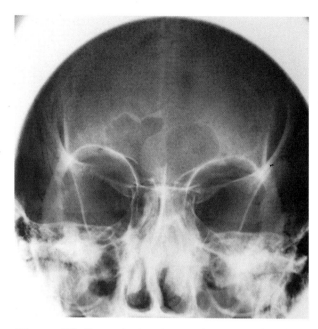

Figure 76 Frontal sinusitis with mucocele. Plain skull X-ray shows loss of lucency of the right frontal sinus, the margins of which have lost their normal irregularity and become thinned

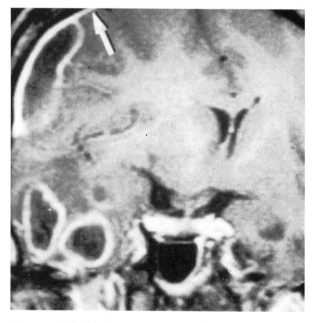

Figure 77 Subdural empyema. This enhanced CT shows two ring-enhancing lesions with a lower-density center in the right temporal region. There is a larger extra-axial collection lying superiorly. The margins are enhanced and the center is of low density. The lower lesions are abscess cavities whereas the uppermost lesion is a subdural empyema

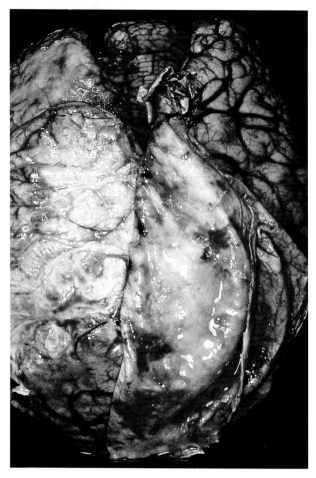

Figure 78 Subdural empyema. A 42-year-old man was admitted to hospital with a 5-day history of headache, confusion, left facial twitching and swelling of the right temporoparietal scalp. Examination revealed dysarthria, deviation of eyes and head to the left, and left facial focal motor seizures. There was also spasm of the right temporalis and masseter muscles, and a boggy swelling over the right temporal region. Despite surgical intervention and broad-spectrum antibiotics, death ensued 6 days later. In this view of the brain from above, the dura has been reflected from over the right cerebral hemisphere. There is pus adhering to the inner aspect of the dura as well as covering the right cerebral convexity

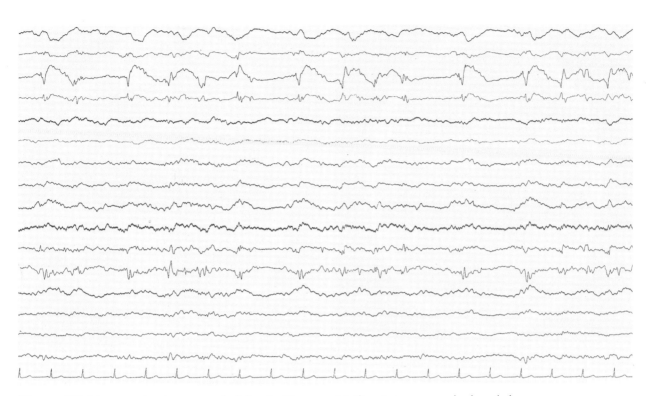

Figure 79 Herpes simplex encephalitis. A 62-year-old Cypriot woman had a 4-day history of headache, fever and deterioration of level of consciousness, and two secondarily generalized tonic-clonic seizures. EEG shows 'periodic complexes' – high-voltage sharp waves occurring at 2-s intervals over the right posterior temporal region. From top to bottom: Fp2–F8, F8–T4, T4–T6, T6–02; Fp1–F7, F7–T3, T3–T5, T5–01; Fp2–F4, F4–C4, C4–P4, P4–02; Fp1–F3, F3–C3, C3–P3 and P3–01

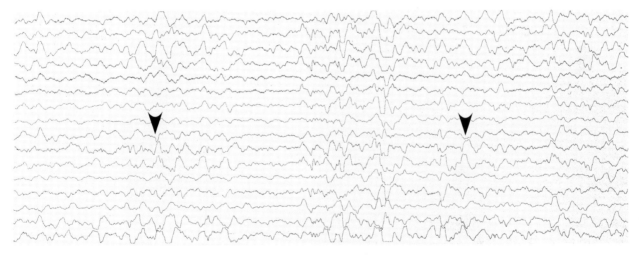

Figure 80 Herpes simplex encephalitis. A 7-year-old boy had focal seizures and increasing stupor due to herpes simplex encephalitis. EEG shows bilateral but asymmetrical high-amplitude paroxysmal activity against a slow background. The slow activity predominates over the left hemisphere (arrowed) whereas the right is of relatively low amplitude. From top to bottom: Fp2–T4, T4–02; Fp1–T3, T3–01; Fp2–F4, F4–C4, C4–P4, P4–02; Fp1–F3, F3–C3, C3–P3, P3–01; T4–C4, C4–Cz, Cz–C3 and C3–T3

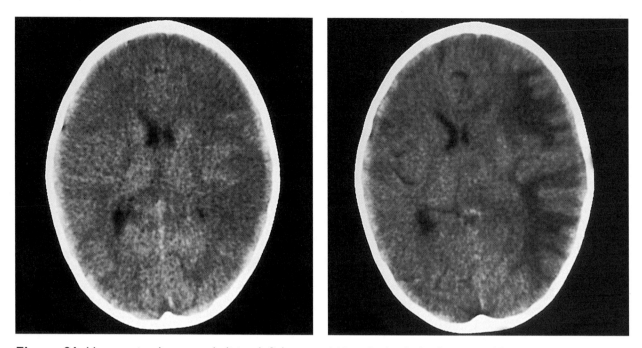

Figure 81 Herpes simplex encephalitis. A 2¹/₂-year-old boy had a 3-day history of frequent partial and generalized seizures and eventual coma due to herpes simplex encephalitis. Axial CT shows initially a diffuse loss of white–gray matter differentiation and low densities bilaterally, particularly in the right temporoparietal region (left); 10 days later, there was diffuse infarction of the right hemisphere (right)

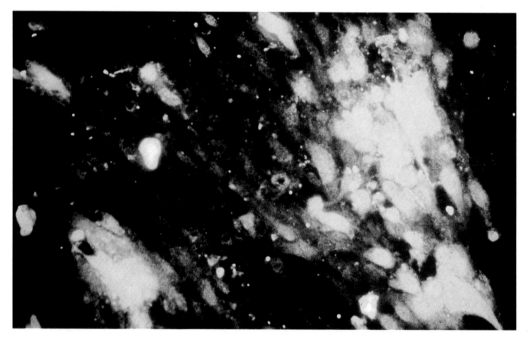

Figure 82 Herpes simplex encephalitis. Immunofluorescence of the temporal lobe reveals the presence of fluorescent-labelled antibody and, therefore, abundant herpes simplex antigen. This is one of many reliable methods for diagnosing herpes simplex infection of brain tissue

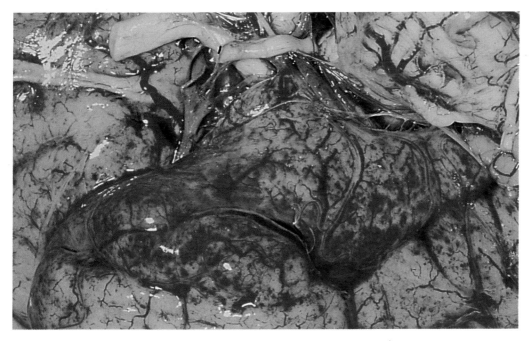

Figure 83 Herpes simplex encephalitis. The base of the right brain shows an area of hemorrhagic necrosis affecting the right uncus and adjacent parts of the temporal lobe. This location and appearance are typical of acute herpes simplex encephalitis

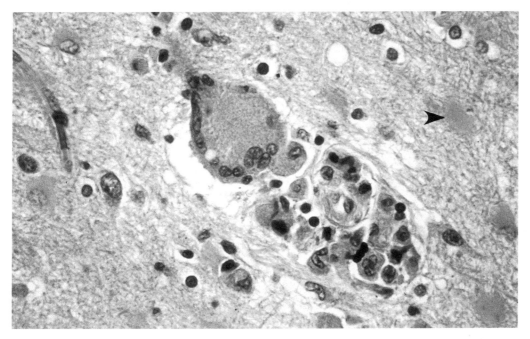

Figure 84 HIV encephalitis in AIDS. Histology shows perivascular clusters of virus-infected cells of the monocyte–macrophage series, some of which are multinucleated. There is also evidence of white matter gliosis with gemistocytic astrocytes (arrowed) and demyelination. (H & E)

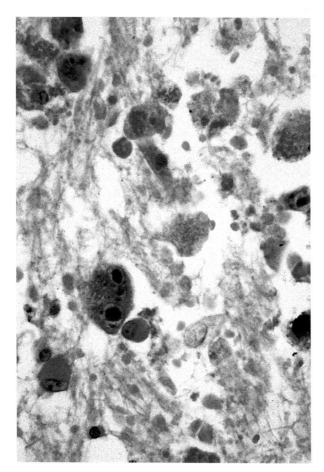 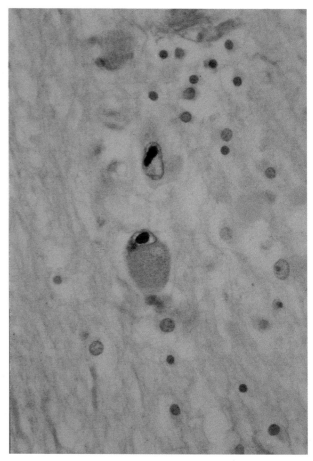

Figure 85 Cytomegalovirus encephalitis in AIDS. The presence of conspicuous intranuclear inclusions of viral material in enlarged virus-infected cells characterizes this pathological entity. (H & E)

Figure 86 Cytomegalovirus encephalitis in AIDS. Immunohistochemistry for cytomegalovirus antigen confirms its presence within the nuclei of infected cells

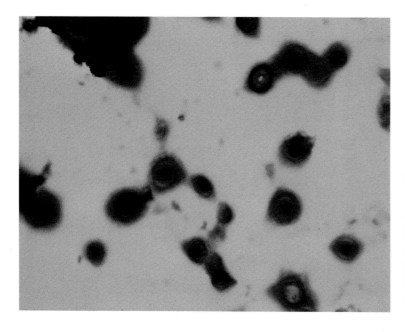

Figure 87 Cryptococcal meningitis in AIDS. Cryptococcal meningitis is characterized by a diffuse growth of organisms within the meninges with a minimal associated inflammation. The yeasts are readily identifiable by their metachromatic mucoid capsules. (Toluidine blue)

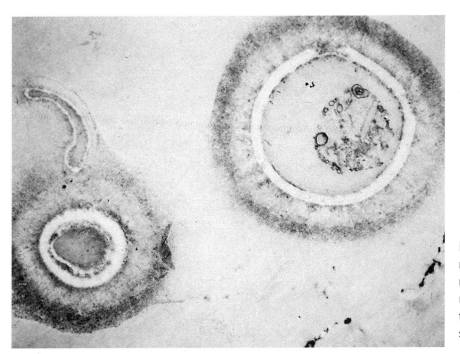

Figure 88 Cryptococcal meningitis in AIDS. Electron microscopy of *Cryptococcus* reveals their ultrastructure; the mucoid capsule is readily seen

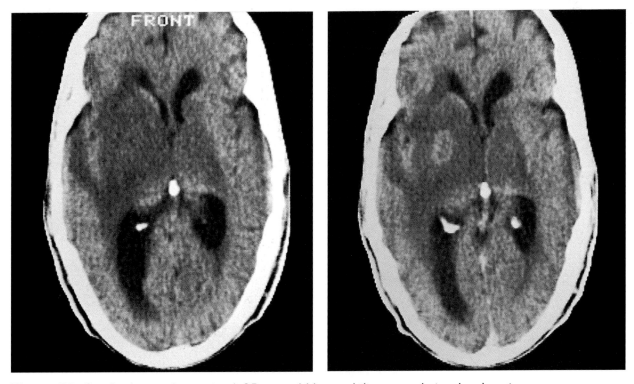

Figure 89 Cerebral toxoplasmosis. A 35-year-old hemophiliac was admitted to hospital in a postictal confusional state. Examination revealed a dense right hemiparesis. CTs reveal extensive low-density change deep within the left hemisphere involving the thalamus, head of the caudate, internal capsule and putamen. Within this lies an enhancing area with a slightly denser rim, suggestive of the presence of an abscess cavity. The patient recovered fully with appropriate treatment

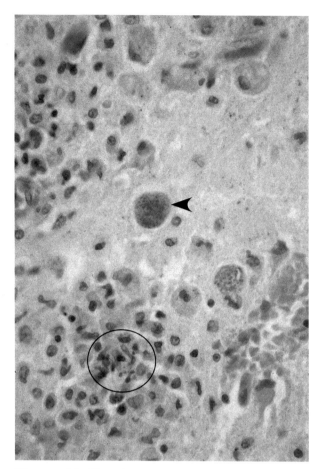

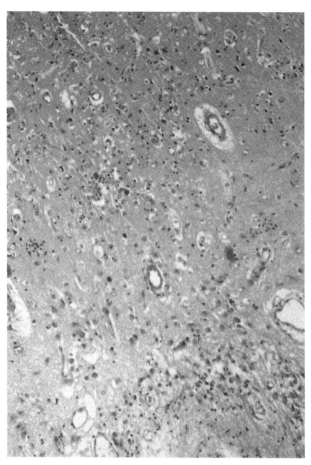

Figure 90 *Toxoplasma* encephalitis in AIDS. Histology shows extensive mononuclear inflammation together with the presence of several pseudocysts containing bradyzoites (arrowed); free tachyzoites can also be seen in the tissues (encircled). (H & E)

Figure 91 *Toxoplasma* abscess. A 25-year-old male homosexual presented in a comatose state with neck stiffness and seizures. This was treated as bacterial meningitis; death ensued 3 days later. Histology of the cerebral cortex shows focal encephalitic lesions. (H & E; see Figure 92)

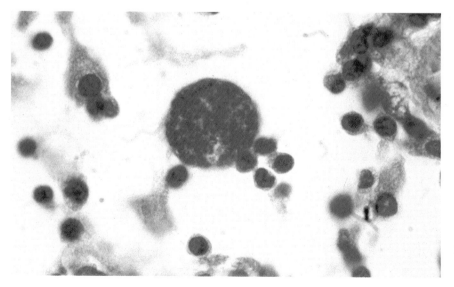

Figure 92 *Toxoplasma* abscess. Histology shows a pseudocyst filled with bradyzoites of *Toxoplasma gondii*. (H & E)

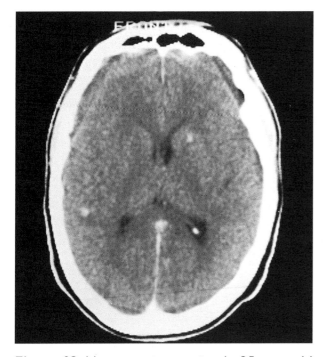

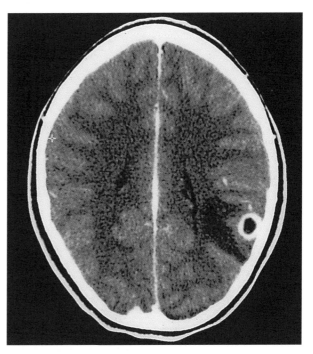

Figure 93 Neurocysticercosis. A 35-year-old doctor working for the World Health Organization had travelled throughout many underdeveloped countries, including both Central America and India. He had a history of occasional nocturnal tonic-clonic seizures and some daytime episodes suggestive of temporal lobe onset. Non-enhanced CT shows small areas of hyperdensity (calcium density) scattered throughout both hemispheres

Figure 94 Neurocysticercosis. A 7-year-old boy from Pakistan had a 2-month history of recurrent partial seizures, headache and low-grade fever due to infestation with *Taenia solium* (neurocysticercosis). Contrast-enhanced axial CT shows a single ring-enhancing lesion with surrounding edema in the left parietal lobe

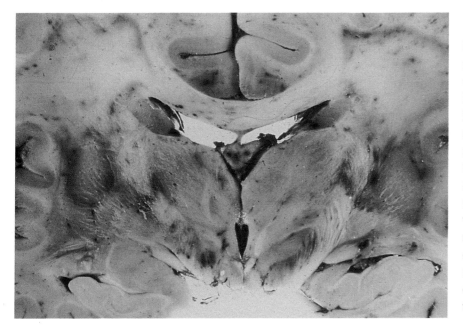

Figure 95 Cerebral malaria. Coronal section through the cerebrum at the level of the mammillary bodies shows the typical appearances of fatal malaria due to *Plasmodium falciparum*. There is generalized edema. The numerous petechial hemorrhages, most evident in the white matter of the centrum semiovale and the internal capsules, represent hemorrhage around small vessels occluded by parasitized erythrocytes

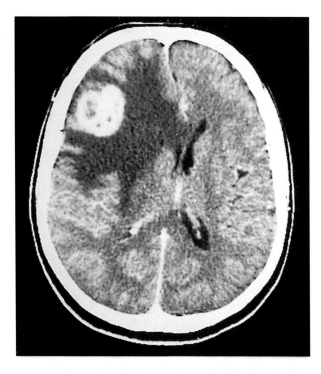

Figure 96 Tuberculoma. A 45-year-old Egyptian woman presented with a 3-month history of headache and mild confusion. CT demonstrates a hyperdense lesion in the right frontal region with surrounding low-density edema and mass effect. The patient underwent a diagnostic craniotomy

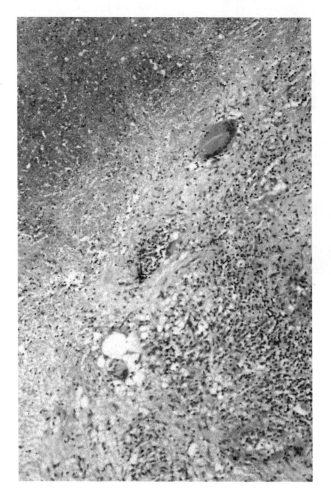

Figure 97 Tuberculoma. Histology of the wall of a cerebral tuberculoma shows extensive coagulative necrosis with an adjacent inflammatory reaction, characterized by fibrosis and infiltration by lymphocytes, epithelioid cells and Langerhans' giant cells. (H & E)

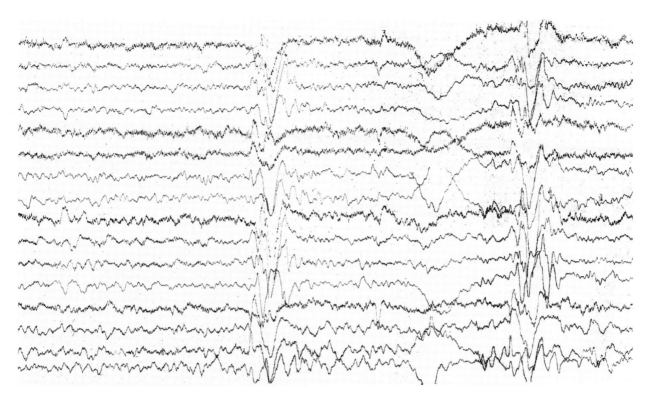

Figure 98 Subacute sclerosing panencephalitis. EEG of a 7-year-old boy with subacute sclerosing panencephalitis shows paroxysmal high-amplitude slow-wave complexes that recur periodically unaccompanied by clinical change

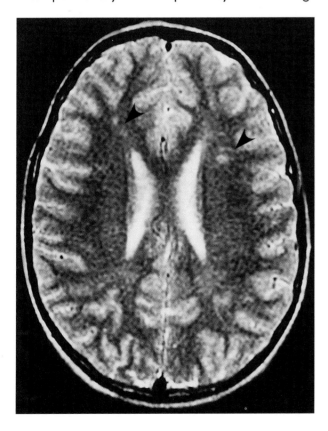

Figure 99 Subacute sclerosing panencephalitis. A 13-year-old boy had a history of altered behavior, declining school performance and infrequent generalized tonic-clonic seizures due to subacute sclerosing panencephalitis. T_2-weighted MRI shows areas of high signal in the periventricular white matter (arrowed) which are indicative of demyelination

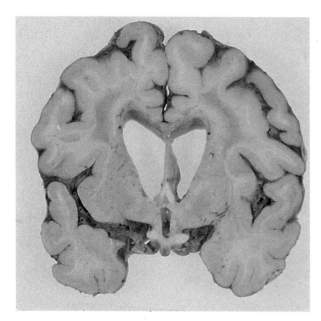

Figure 100 Subacute sclerosing panencephalitis. Coronal section of the cerebrum at the level of the optic chiasm shows generalized cerebral atrophy with dilatation of the lateral and third ventricles. The cerebral white matter has been reduced in bulk and shows gray discoloration due to the presence of diffuse gliosis

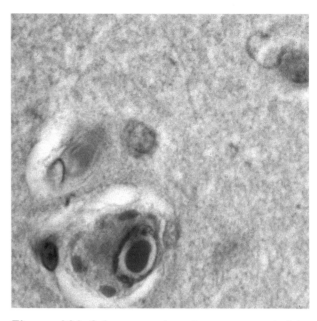

Figure 101 Subacute sclerosing panencephalitis. Histology of the cerebral cortex shows several large intranuclear inclusions of measles virus. (H & E)

Figure 102 Neurosyphilis. A 36-year-old homo-sexual hairdresser was admitted to hospital on three occasions with secondarily generalized tonic-clonic seizures. On the third occasion, he was transferred to the neurology unit in a confusional state. EEG (top of facing page) revealed periodic lateralized epileptiform discharges (PLEDs) on a generally slow background, appearances interpreted as complex partial status epilepticus. From top to bottom: Fp2–F8, F8–T4, T4–T6, T6–02; Fp2–F4, F4–C4, C4–P4, P4–02; Fp1–F7, F7–T3, T3–T5, T5–01; Fp1–F3, F3–C3, C3–P3 and P3–01.

Despite resolution of his non-convulsive status, his mental state remained abnormal. Serological tests in blood and cerebrospinal fluid suggested active neurosyphilis. After treatment with procaine penicillin and prednisolone, psychometry revealed an IQ of 70 with profound verbal and visual memory deficits. Six months later, he was functioning well at work; at that time, blood and cerebrospinal fluid rapid plasma reagin was negative

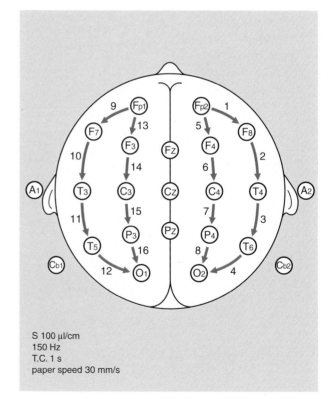

S 100 μl/cm
150 Hz
T.C. 1 s
paper speed 30 mm/s

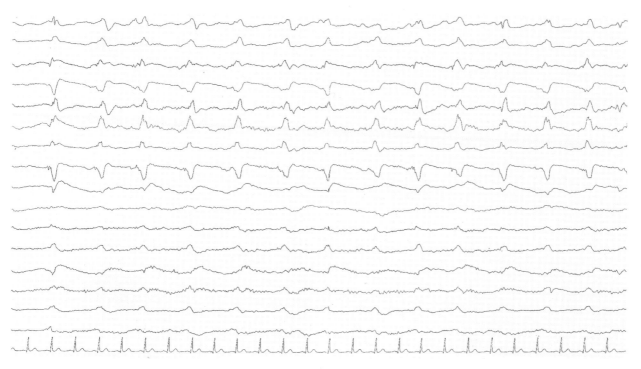

Figure 102 continued From top to bottom: Fp2–F4, F4–C4, C4–P4, P4–02; Fp1–F3, F3–C3, C3–P3, P3–01; Fp2–F8, F8–T4, T4–T6, T6–02; Fp1–F7, F7–T3, T3–T5 and T5–01

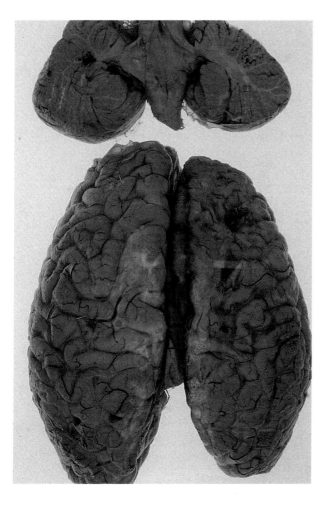

Figure 103 Neurosyphilis. Gross appearances of cerebellum and brain stem (upper), and cerebrum (lower) viewed from above, show changes mainly of meningovascular syphilis with diffuse leptomeningeal thickening. There are multiple areas of cortical infarction particularly in the right hemisphere secondary to endarteritis obliterans of the meningeal arteries

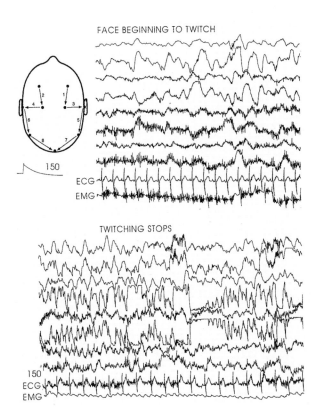

FACE BEGINNING TO TWITCH

ECG
EMG

TWITCHING STOPS

150
ECG
EMG

Figure 104 Rasmussen's 'encephalitis'. This 4-year-old boy had an 8-month history of increasingly frequent right-sided myoclonic and clonic seizures affecting the face and arm, with secondarily generalized tonic-clonic seizures and episodes of convulsive status epilepticus. EEG shows virtually continuous slow-wave activity in the left frontal region with build-up to a prolonged run of discharges in the frontal and central regions associated with a seizure. The patient developed a progressive right hemiparesis and dysphasia

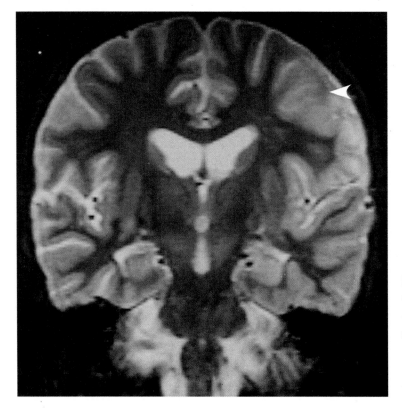

Figure 105 Rasmussen's 'encephalitis'. Coronal MRI (same patient as in Figure 104) demonstrates a high-signal and thickened cortex in the left posterior frontal region (arrowed). Brain biopsy of the cortical abnormality confirmed the diagnosis

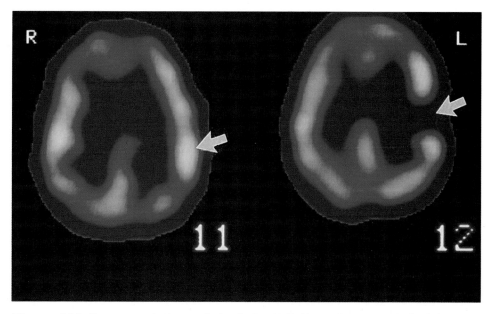

Figure 106 Rasmussen's 'encephalitis'. Ictal (left) and interictal (right) technetium-99-labelled HMPAO-SPECT scans (same patient as in Figures 104 and 105) show a focal area of hyperperfusion and hypoperfusion, respectively, in the left posterior frontal region (arrowed). Intravenous methylprednisolone and immunoglobulins were ineffective. Hemispherectomy was undertaken 4 years and 3 months after diagnosis

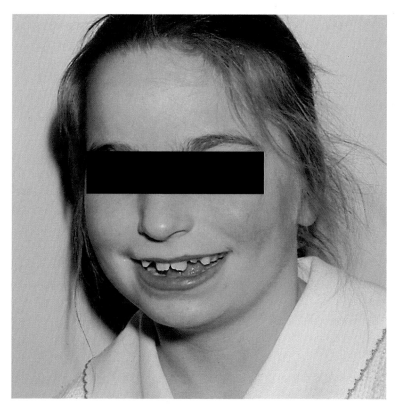

Figure 107 Angelman's syndrome. An 8-year-old girl with this syndrome (left) experienced tonic and myoclonic-atonic seizures. EEGs (overleaf) show runs of slow 3-cps waves which are frequently notched (arrowed) and occasionally associated with true spikes

Figure 107 continued From top to bottom: Fp2–F4, F4–C4, C4–P4, P4–02; Fp1–F3, F3–C3, C3–P3, P3–01; Fp2–F8, F8–T4, T4–T6, T6–02; Fp1–F7, F7–T3, T3–T5 and T5–01

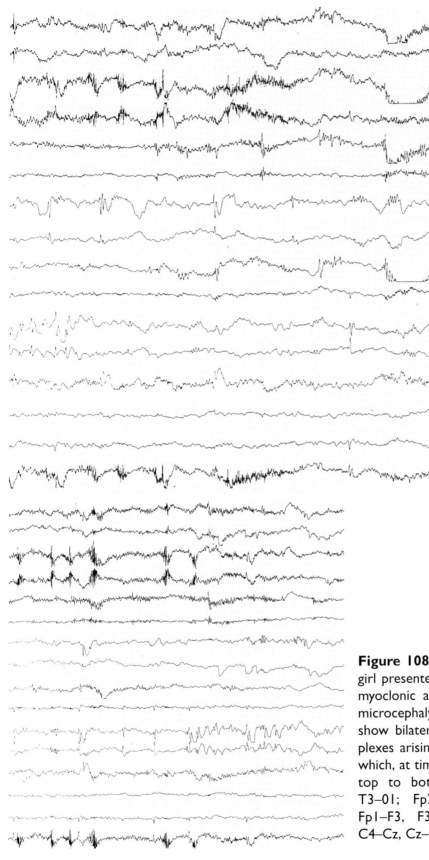

Figure 108 Rett syndrome. A 21-month-old girl presented with developmental regression, myoclonic and atonic seizures, and acquired microcephaly due to Rett syndrome. EEGs show bilateral independent spike–wave complexes arising from posterior regions (upper) which, at times, occur in bursts (lower). From top to bottom: Fp2–T4, T4–02; Fp1–T3, T3–01; Fp2–F4, F4–C4, C4–P4, P4–02; Fp1–F3, F3–C3, C3–P3, P3–01; T4–C4, C4–Cz, Cz–C3 and C3–T3

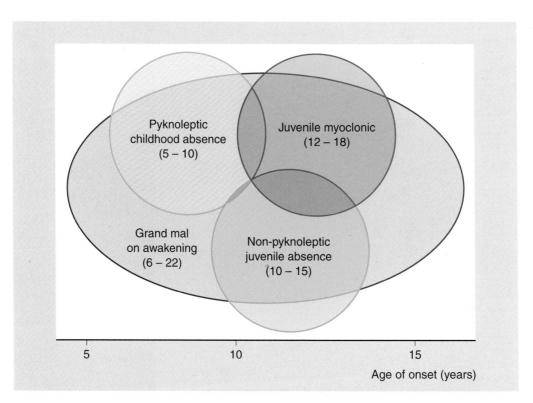

Age of onset (years)

Figure 109 Age of onset and overlap of the different epilepsy syndromes within the category of primary idiopathic generalized epilepsy (IGE). With permission, from Janz D. Juvenile myoclonic epilepsy. In: Dam M, Gram L, eds. *Comprehensive Epileptology*. New York: Raven Press, 1990:171–85

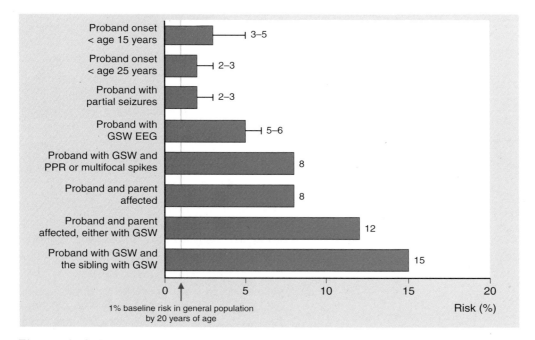

Figure 110 Sibling risk for epilepsy. GSW, generalized spike and wave; PPR, photoparoxysmal response. With permission, from Laidlaw J, Richens A, Chadwick D, eds. *A Textbook of Epilepsy*, 4th edn. London: Churchill Livingstone, 1993:64

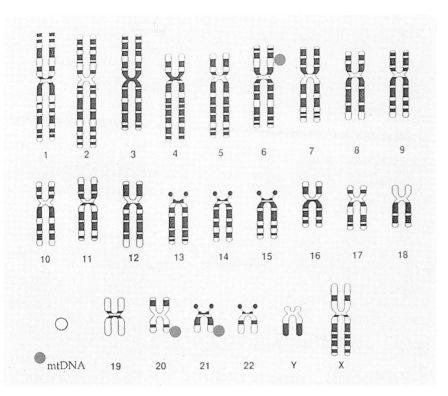

Figure 111 Human karyotype. The red spots indicate the first three chromosomes which are relevant to epilepsy syndromes

Mendelian epilepsy gene map (autosomal)

Dominantly inherited conditions

Epilepsy locus	Location	Gene product
Tuberous sclerosis complex 1	9q 3.4	–
Tuberous sclerosis complex 2	16p 13	tuberin
Neurofibromatosis 1	17q 11.2	neurofibromin
Huntington's disease	4p 16	Huntingtin
Miller–Dieker syndrome	17p	–
Benign neonatal familial convulsions	20q	?CHRNA4
Benign neonatal familial convulsions	8q	–
Partial epilepsies	10q 2.3	–
Autosomal dominant nocturnal frontal lobe epilepsy	20q	CHRNA4

Recessively inherited conditions

Epilepsy locus	Location	Gene product
Unverricht–Lundborg disease	21q 22	Cystatin B
Infantile neuronal ceroid lipofuscinosis	1p	palmitoyl protein thioesterase
Juvenile neuronal ceroid lipofuscinosis	16p	438 amino acids
Lafora's body disease	6q	–
Northern epilepsy	8p	–

Figure 112 Mendelian epilepsy gene map. These 14 conditions have been linked to specific chromosomes. In most instances, the gene product has been identified

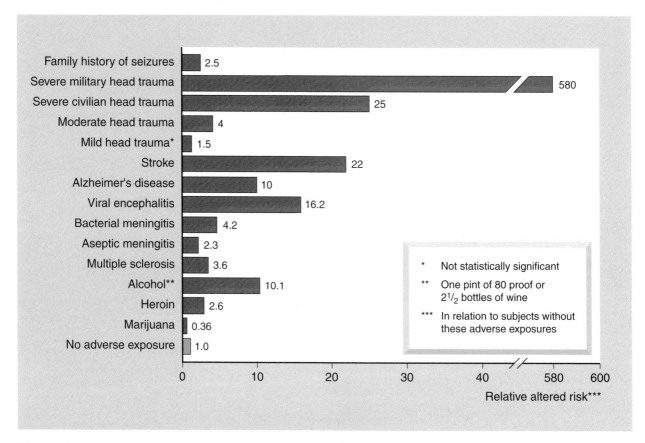

Figure 113 Risk of epilepsy associated with various cerebral insults

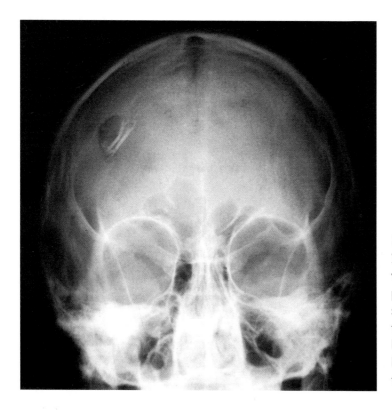

Figure 114 Depressed skull fracture. A 21-year-old man was struck on the head with a hammer and was admitted to hospital in generalized convulsive status. Plain skull X-ray shows a depressed fracture in the left parietal region close to the midline. The fracture is comminuted and two large fragments are depressed well into the brain

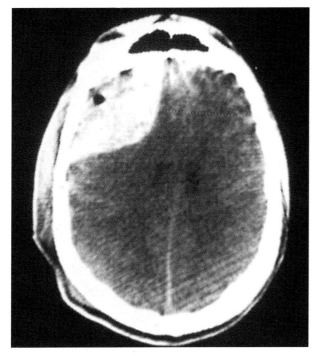

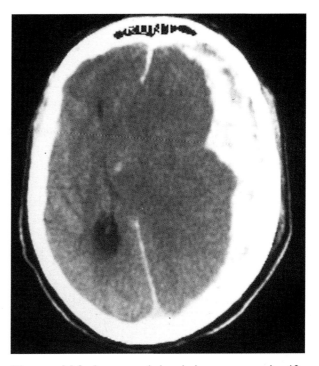

Figure 115 Extradural hematoma. A 30-year-old man was knocked off his motorbike in a road traffic accident. He was comatose with a right hemiparesis and right-sided hemiconvulsions. CT shows a large hyperdense lens-shaped extradural hematoma in the extradural space of the left frontal and temporal regions. The latter contains a small quantity of air

Figure 116 Acute subdural hematoma. A 40-year-old man sustained multiple injuries when he fell from a second-storey window. CT reveals an extensive hyperdense acute subdural hematoma which overlies the surface of the brain and follows the curve of the inner table

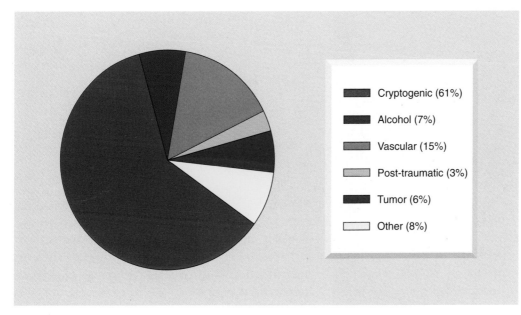

Figure 117 Etiology of newly diagnosed epilepsy

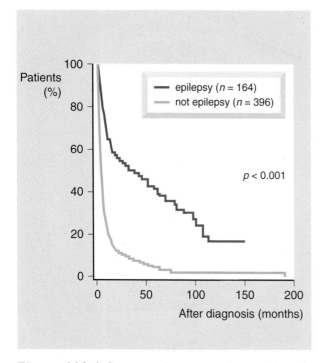

Figure 118 Influence of presentation with epilepsy on survival experience of patients with cerebral tumors

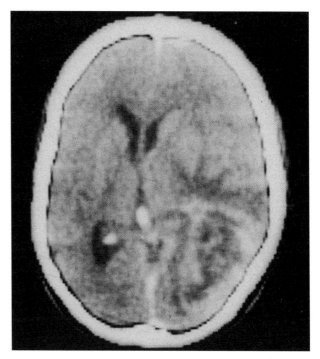

Figure 119 Glioblastoma multiforme. A 51-year-old man gave a 2-month history of headache and visual disturbance. He then experienced a single witnessed generalized tonic-clonic seizure. Examination revealed a left homonymous hemianopia and papilledema. Contrast-enhanced CT shows an irregular mass in the right occipital region with surrounding edema. The wall shows enhancement, but the center is low density and may be necrotic

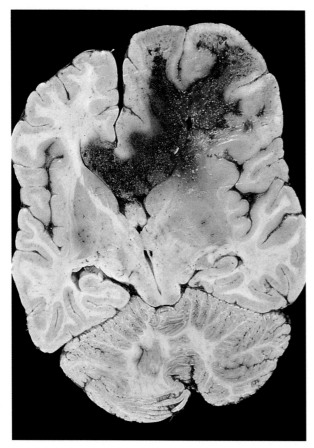

Figure 120 Glioblastoma multiforme. Horizontal section of the brain shows a large glioblastoma involving much of the right frontal lobe and extending into the opposite hemisphere through the corpus callosum. Much of the tumor has undergone hemorrhagic necrosis, but a rim of viable tumor is identifiable diffusely infiltrating the structures of the right frontal pole

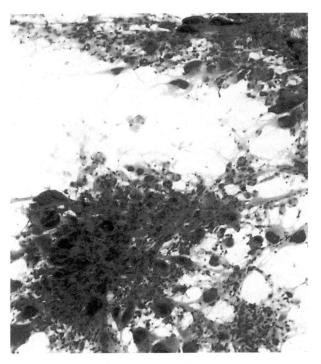

Figure 121 Glioblastoma multiforme. Smear preparation of a glioblastoma reveals the characteristic pleomorphic population of poorly differentiated astrocytes. (H & E)

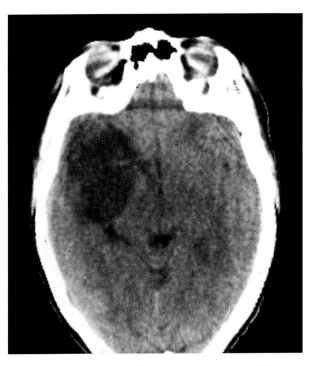

Figure 122 Low-grade astrocytoma. A 35-year-old woman had a history of somatosensory auras and occasional olfactory hallucinations. She also had a history of intermittent psychotic behavior. Her initial neurological examination was normal, but she developed a mild expressive dysphasia. CT shows a lesion of mixed signal intensity with an associated mass effect in the left temporoparietal region

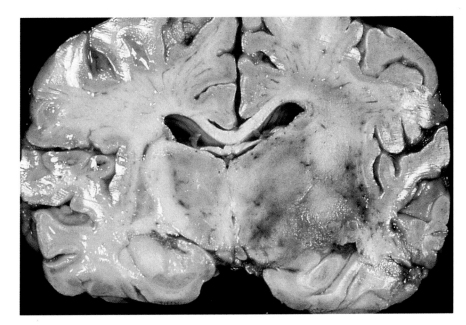

Figure 123 Low-grade astrocytoma. Coronal section at the level of the mammillary bodies shows an extensive, diffusely infiltrating, neoplasm in the right hemisphere effacing the basal ganglia, thalamus and surrounding structures

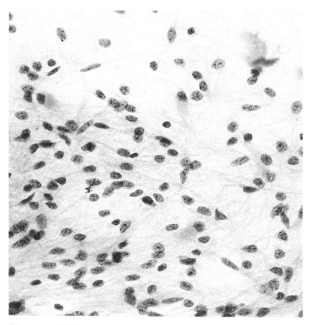

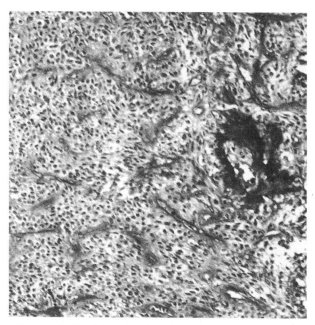

Figure 124 Low-grade astrocytoma. Smear preparation reveals a diffuse growth of well-differentiated astrocytes often forming conspicuous fibrillary processes. (H & E)

Figure 125 Oligodendroglioma. Histology typically shows a diffuse growth of small rounded cells with an intricate capillary network and foci of calcification. (H & E)

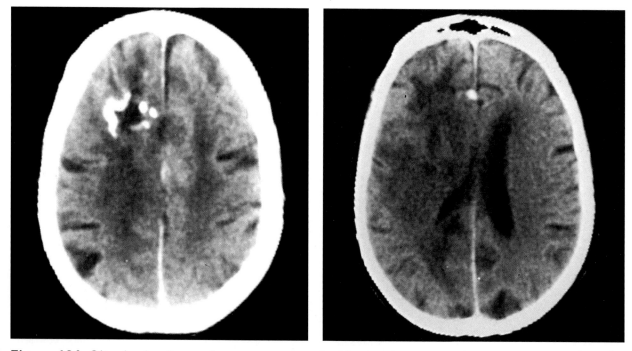

Figure 126 Oligodendroglioma. A woman presented with partial seizures in her midforties. Epilepsy was the only manifestation for 10 years but, thereafter, she deteriorated progressively with increasing fit frequency, progressive cognitive decline and a right hemiparesis. CTs show a zone of calcification in the left frontal region, with surrounding low density and mass effect

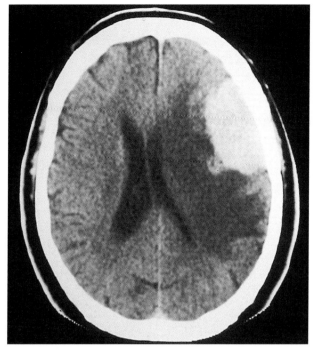

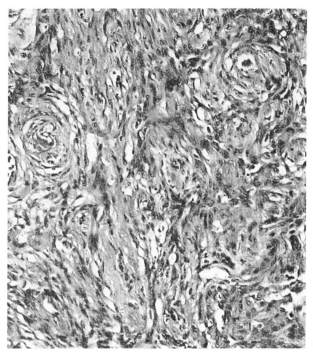

Figure 127 Meningioma. A 57-year-old man presented with right facial focal motor seizures and a gradually progressive dysphasia. Enhanced CT shows a large hyperdense, slightly lobulated mass attached to the convexity in the left posterior frontal region. There is surrounding edema with compression of the left lateral ventricle and some midline shift

Figure 128 Meningioma. Histology consists of well-differentiated meningothelial (arachnoidal) cells growing in sheets and whorls. (H & E)

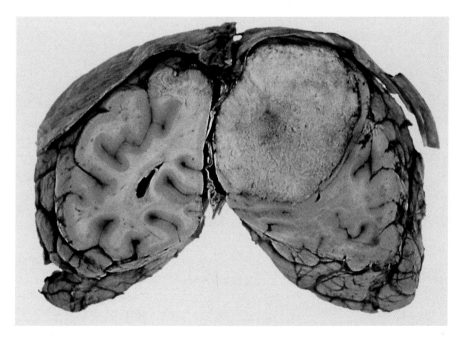

Figure 129 Meningioma. Coronal section of cerebrum in parieto-occipital region shows a typically well demarcated meningioma attached to, but not invading, the underlying brain

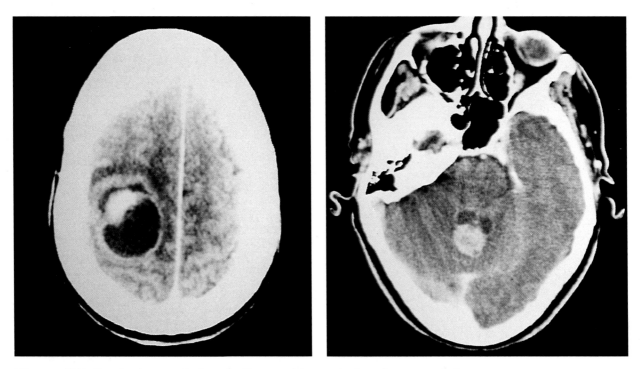

Figure 130 Cerebral secondaries. A 60-year-old man had undergone a left pneumonectomy for bronchial carcinoma at the age of 54. He presented with truncal ataxia, focal motor seizures and progressive left-arm weakness. CTs show an enhancing area within the vermis causing slight distortion of the fourth ventricle. There is also an area of ring-shaped enhancement in the right parietal region with a cystic component

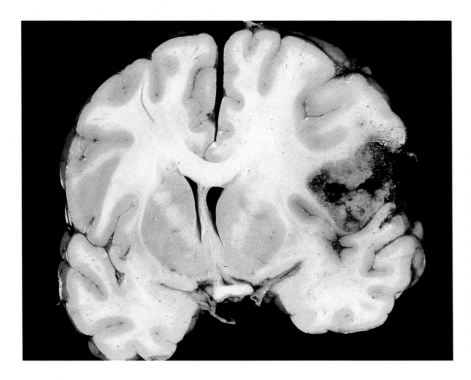

Figure 131 Cerebral secondaries. Coronal section of cerebrum at the level of the optic chiasm shows a well-defined intrinsic tumor with central necrosis. Cystic degeneration is present immediately above the right sylvian fissure. Carcinomas are characteristically well demarcated from the adjacent brain tissue

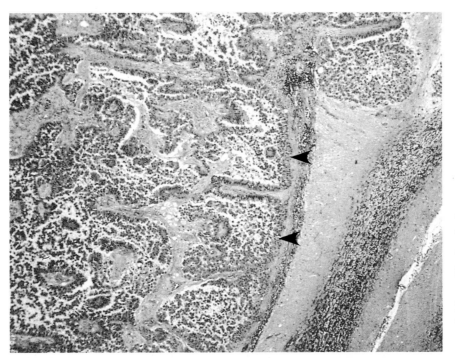

Figure 132 Cerebral secondaries. Histology of a metastatic adenocarcinoma in the cerebellum shows the disorganized papillary processes (arrowed) to be well differentiated from the surviving cerebellar cortical tissue. (H & E)

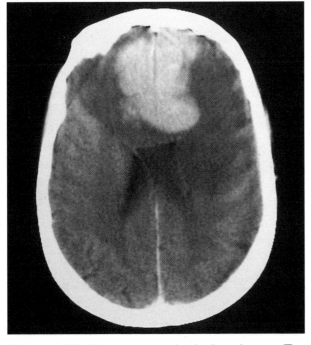

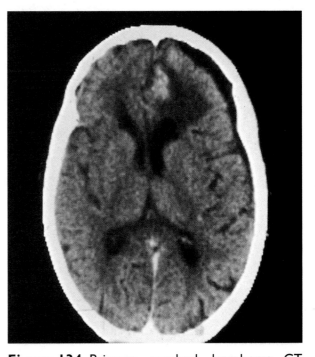

Figure 133 Primary cerebral lymphoma. Ten years after a successful renal transplant, a 37-year-old man developed early morning headaches and vomiting. He was admitted to hospital after a single tonic-clonic seizure and became comatose with papilledema. CT shows a homogeneously enhancing mass in the right frontal region with extensive surrounding edema

Figure 134 Primary cerebral lymphoma. CT (same patient as in **Figure 133**) after diagnostic biopsy and steroid treatment shows that the volume of the mass has greatly diminished and the edema has virtually resolved

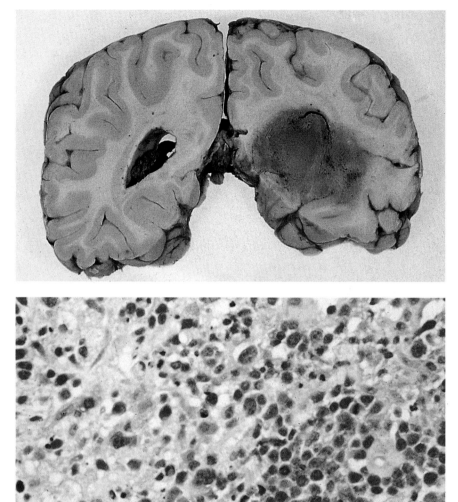

Figure 135 Primary cerebral lymphoma. Coronal section of cerebrum immediately posterior to the corpus callosum splenium shows an ill-defined diffusely infiltrating tumor adjacent to the right lateral ventricle. Primary cerebral lymphomas are often multiple, periventricular and ill-defined

Figure 136 Primary cerebral lymphoma. Histology reveals that these are nearly always high-grade non-Hodgkin's B-cell lymphomas. They diffusely infiltrate the brain, but show accentuation of infiltration around blood vessels. (H & E)

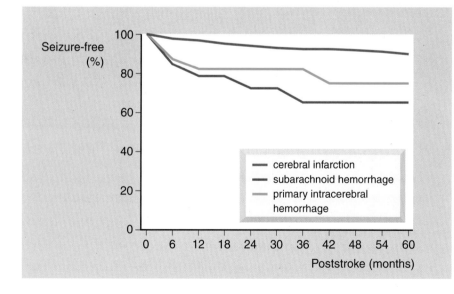

Figure 137 Risks of seizure after stroke. Modified from Burn J, Sandercock P, Bamford J, *et al.* Epileptic seizures after first ever in a lifetime stroke. The Oxfordshire Community Stroke Project. *Br Med J* 1997

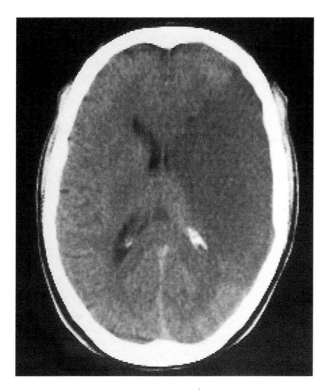

Figure 138 Cerebral infarction. A 64-year-old man presented with a single generalized tonic-clonic seizure. Examination revealed weakness of the left arm and face. CT shows a large infarction in the left middle cerebral artery territory. With treatment, the patient experiences occasional focal motor seizures

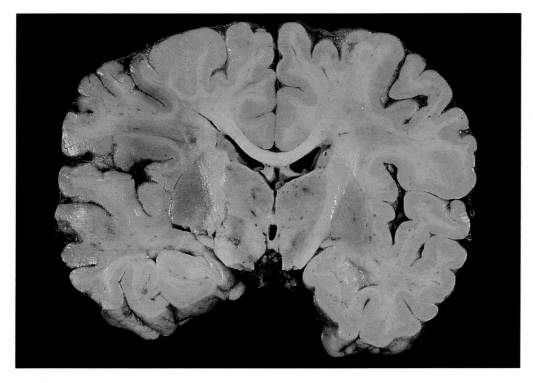

Figure 139 Recent cerebral infarct (ischemic). Coronal section of cerebrum shows the presence of a recent infarct in the left middle cerebral artery territory characterized by diffuse edema with blurring of the junction between gray and white matter

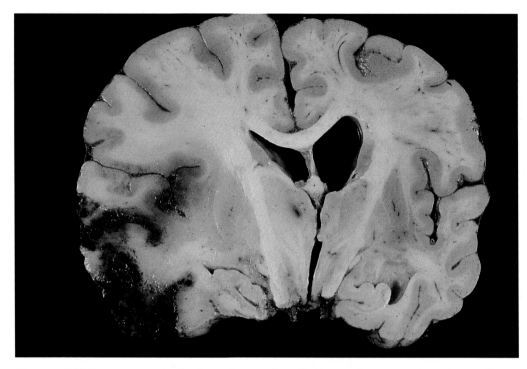

Figure 140 Recent cerebral infarct (hemorrhagic). Coronal section of cerebrum shows the presence of a recent hemorrhagic infarct in the overlap zone between the middle cerebral and posterior cerebral artery territories characterized by hemorrhage, most obvious in the gray matter. There is white matter edema, blurring of gray–white matter differentiation and conspicuous shift of midline structures from left to right, with ventricular compression and ipsilateral tentorial herniation. Hemorrhagic infarcts are due to the reestablishment of perfusion through devitalized brain tissue and may also be due to, for example, transient cerebral hypoperfusion or lysis of an embolus previously occluding a supplying artery

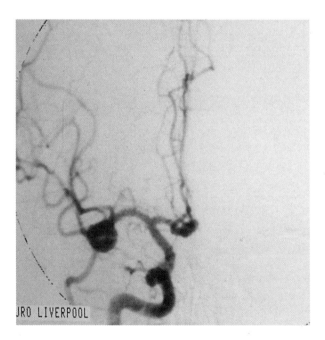

Figure 141 Middle cerebral artery aneurysm. Five days prior to hospital admission, a 68-year-old man developed a sudden severe headache and vomited. Physical examination and CT were normal, but cerebrospinal fluid was xanthochromic, and angiography revealed a large middle cerebral artery aneurysm and smaller right anterior communicating artery aneurysms. Because of his age, the presence of multiple lesions and the increased risk of epilepsy, the patient decided not to undergo surgery

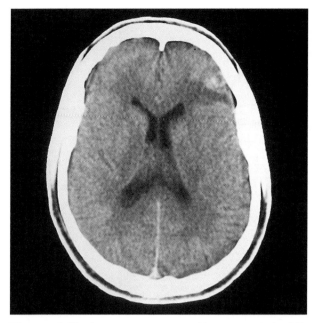

Figure 142 Arteriovenous malformation. A 27-year-old man presented with a 1-month history of headache and two nocturnal tonic-clonic seizures. Physical examination was normal, but contrast-enhanced CT shows a small, partly enhancing, lesion in the left frontal region (see Figure 143)

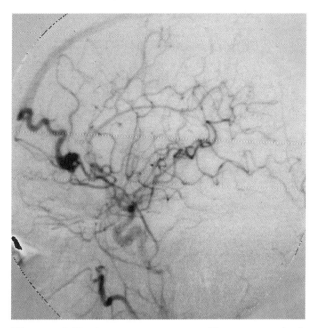

Figure 143 Arteriovenous malformation. Left carotid angiography (same patient as in Figure 142) shows a large feeding vessel arising from the middle cerebral artery. Such a lesion is amenable to focal radiotherapy

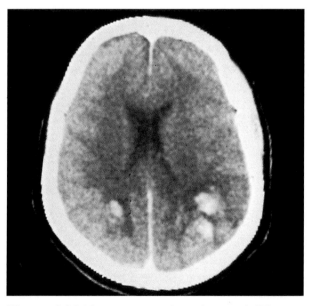

Figure 144 Venous sinus thrombosis. A 30-year-old woman was 2 weeks postpartum when she presented with a 2-day history of headache, seizures and increasing confusion. CT shows hyperdense areas in the occipital lobes of both hemispheres consistent with areas of hemorrhage

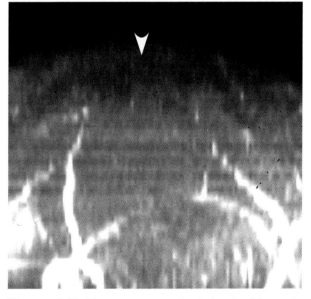

Figure 145 Venous sinus thrombosis. Magnetic resonance venogram (same patient as in Figure 144) shows cortical veins running down from, rather than up towards, the sagittal sinus, which is not patent (arrowed)

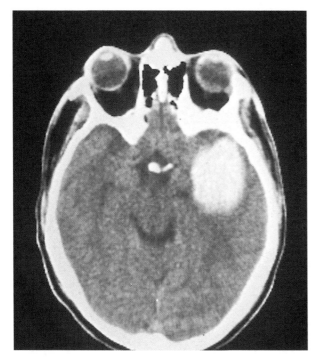

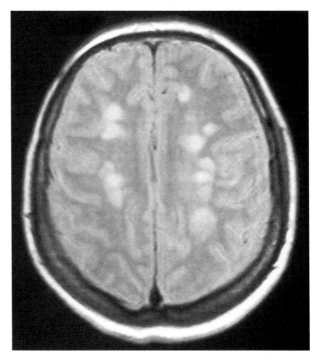

Figure 146 Intracerebral hematoma. A 17-year-old boy presented with an acute onset of headache, vomiting and aphasia. CT shows a hyperdense mass in the left temporal lobe, a small amount of surrounding low-density areas and a mass effect. At craniotomy, no arteriovenous malformation was identified, but a small lesion might have been obliterated by the bleed. Postoperatively, the patient has developed temporal lobe epilepsy

Figure 147 Cerebral lupus. A 49-year-old woman with a clear history of strokes affecting both vertebrobasilar and carotid territories presented with left focal motor seizures that responded to carbamazepine. Extensive vascular screening was normal with the exception of a strongly positive antidouble-stranded DNA antibody (1 : 1280). MRI reveals multiple periventricular high-intensity lesions

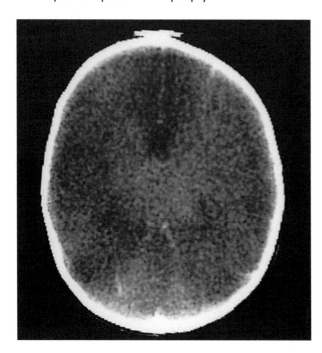

Figure 148 Postcardiac bypass surgery hypoxia. A 9-month-old child had a severe and prolonged hypotensive episode during cardiac bypass surgery and, upon recovery from the anesthetic, was found to be non-responsive and in status epilepticus. Axial CT shows cerebral edema with diffuse areas of low density bilaterally (more on the right than on the left) suggesting cerebral infarction. The patient survived with intractable epilepsy, spastic quadriplegia and cortical visual impairment

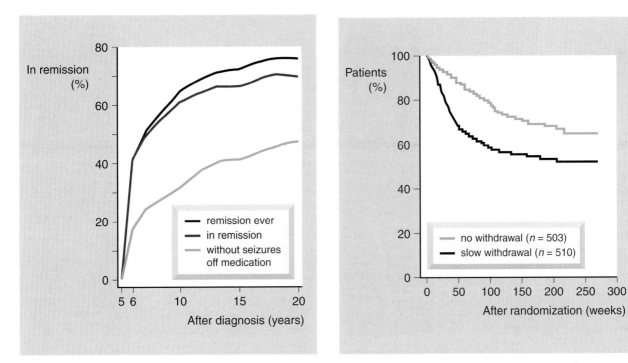

Figure 149 Percentage of patients achieving remission of 5 years or more during the first 20 years after diagnosis of epilepsy

Figure 150 Actuarial percentage of patients remaining seizure-free with continued treatment compared with slow withdrawal of antiepileptic drugs. Modified from reference 7 with permission

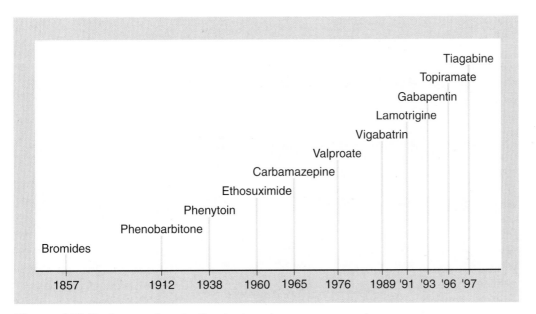

Figure 151 Evolution of antiepileptic drug treatment over time

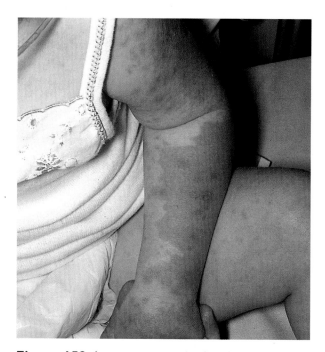

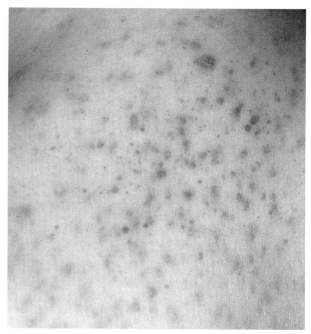

Figure 152 Lamotrigine rash. Six days after lamotrigine was added to her sodium valproate treatment, this 3-year-old girl with myoclonic epilepsy developed a widespread maculopapular rash accompanied by fever, malaise, vomiting and peripheral eosinophilia. The rash resolved within 1 week and recurred when she was 'challenged' with lamotrigine 6 months later

Figure 153 Lamotrigine rash. Five days after lamotrigine was added to his sodium valproate treatment, this 7-year-old boy with Lennox–Gastaut syndrome developed a widespread papular rash associated with low-grade fever which resolved within 10 days

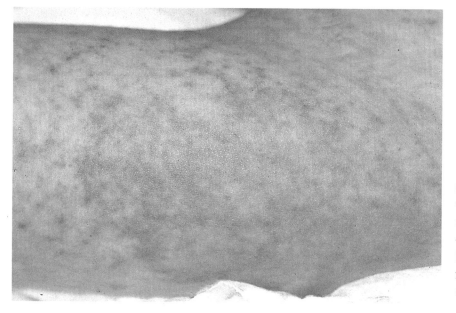

Figure 154 Phenytoin rash. Following a near-drowning accident, an 8-year-old boy was in a coma. A diffuse fine maculopapular rash appeared 48 h after he received a loading dose of phenytoin for seizures. The patient received no other medication

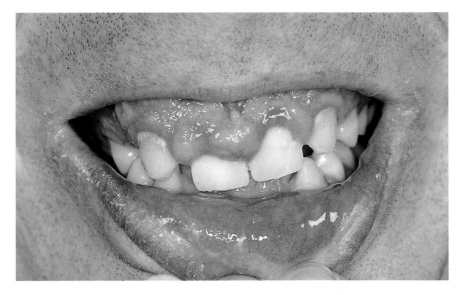

Figure 155 Phenytoin gingival hypertrophy. Moderate gingival hypertrophy has developed in this 32-year-old patient with chronic phenytoin therapy

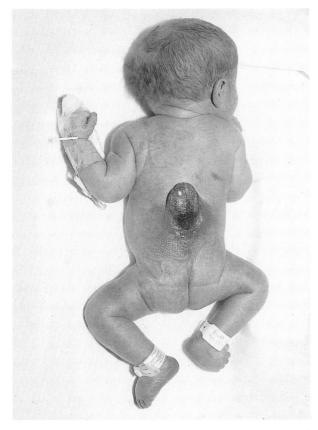

Figure 156 Spina bifida. A mother who had received sodium valproate and carbamazepine during pregnancy gave birth to an infant who had a lower thoracic meningocele with no clinical or radiological evidence of hydrocephalus (ventriculomegaly)

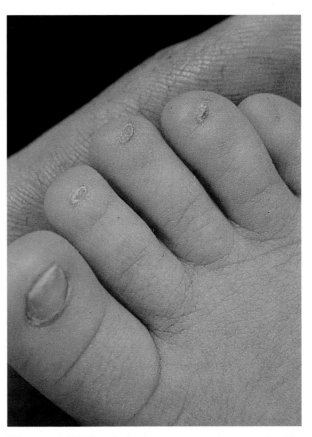

Figure 157 Fetal hydantoin syndrome. A 12-month-old infant, born to a mother with epilepsy who received phenytoin during pregnancy, has hypoplasia of the toenails (as well as of the fingernails), a well-recognized feature of this syndrome

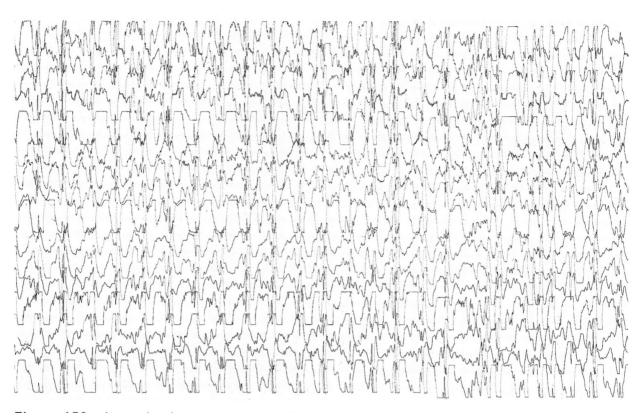

Figure 158 Atypical absence status epilepticus. A 10-year-old boy with Lennox–Gastaut syndrome presented with a 24-h history of confusion, unresponsiveness and semipurposeful movements. Awake EEG shows continuous irregular spike and slow-wave activity. From top to bottom: Fp2–T4, T4–02; Fp1–T3, T3–01; Fp2–F4, F4–C4, C4–P4, P4–02; Fp1–F3, F3–C3, C3–P3, P3–01; T4–C4, C4–Cz, Cz–C3 and C3–T3

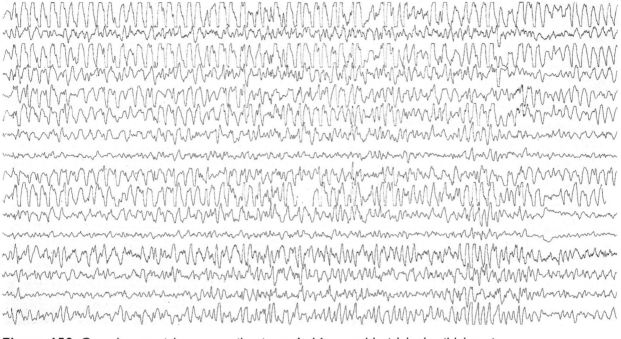

Figure 159 Complex partial status epilepticus. A 16-year-old girl had mild learning difficulties and myoclonic epilepsy. Waking EEG shows virtually continuous spike and slow-wave activity, during which the patient sat unresponsively staring and playing with her clothes, despite the electrical and clinical evidence of complex partial status epilepticus. From top to bottom: Fp2–T4, T4–02; Fp1–T3, T3–01; Fp2–F4, F4–C4, C4–P4, P4–02; Fp1–F3, F3–C3, C3–P3, P3–01; T4–C4, C4–Cz, Cz–C3 and C3–T3

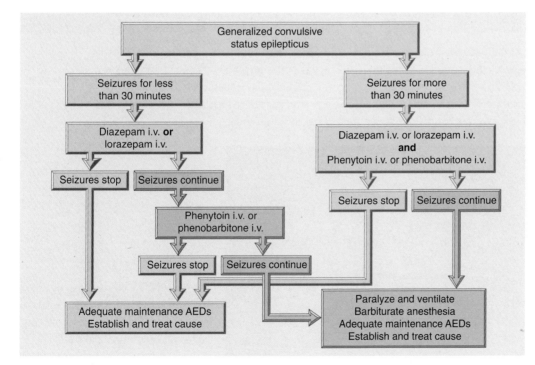

Figure 160 Recommended drug treatment for status epilepticus

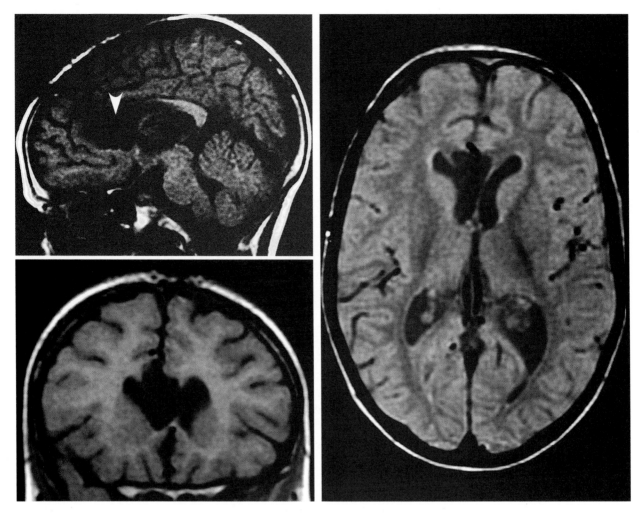

Figure 161 Corpus callosotomy. A 6-year-old boy who had Lennox–Gastaut syndrome experienced daily atonic and tonic sezures that were resistant to antiepileptic drug therapy. Parasagittal (arrowed; upper left), coronal (lower left) and axial (right) MRIs were taken 2 months after sectioning of the anterior two-thirds of the corpus callosum. The atonic and tonic seizures resolved, but the partial seizures increased in frequency

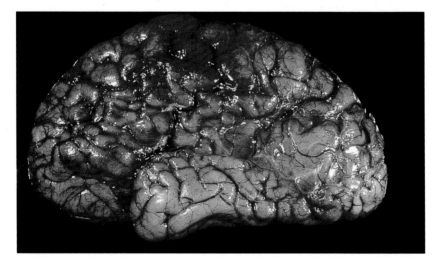

Figure 162 Hemispherectomy. External view of the left cerebral hemisphere shows areas of old ischemic damage particularly in the middle cerebral–posterior cerebral arterial boundary zone

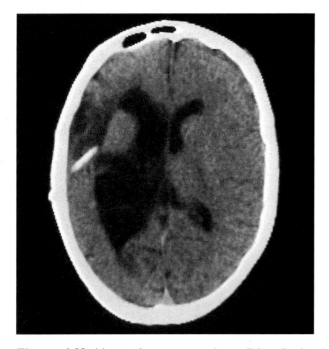

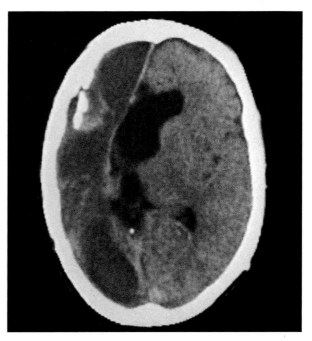

Figure 163 Hemispherectomy. A small boy had a congenital right hemiparesis, and refractory complex partial and secondarily generalized tonic-clonic seizures from the age of 1 year. Preoperative CT shows a shunt in a left temporal arachnoid cyst, left hemisphere atrophy and compensatory hydrocephalus. Postoperatively, he had an intracerebral hemorrhage, disseminated intravascular coagulation and oliguric renal failure

Figure 164 Hemispherectomy. Subsequent CT (same patient as in Figure 163) demonstrates the left hemispherectomy with a low-density collection in the left hemicranium and areas of calcification within this zone, probably representing organization of thrombus. Fortunately, the patient recovered fully and has been seizure-free for at least 2 years; he is able to walk unaided, his verbal communication skills have improved and he has learned to write

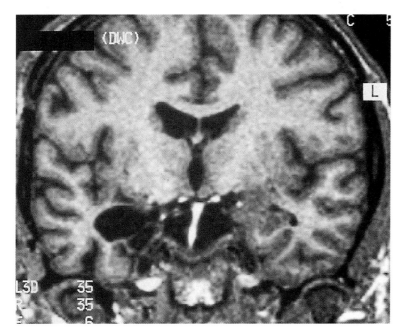

Figure 165 Amygdalohippocampectomy. In a 38-year-old man with refractory temporal lobe seizures, presurgical investigations demonstrated absent right-hemisphere memory function and a right medial temporal seizure onset. Postoperative MRI shows a low-signal area isointense with cerebrospinal fluid, on the medial surface of the right temporal lobe; such changes are typically seen after this operation

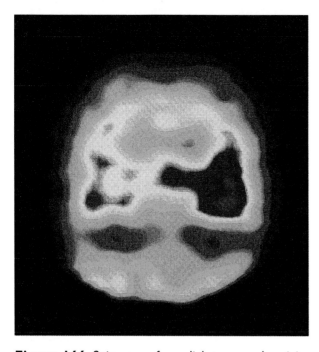

Figure 166 Seizures of medial temporal origin. Ictal HMPAO-SPECT scan shows left temporal hyperperfusion extending into the basal ganglia and adjacent frontal lobe, a typical pattern seen in these seizures

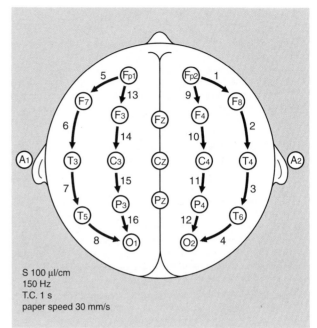

S 100 µl/cm
150 Hz
T.C. 1 s
paper speed 30 mm/s

Figure 167 EEG (below) shows a well-localized interictal right anterior temporal spike focus. From top to bottom: Fp2–F8, F8–T4, T4–T6, T6–02; Fp1–F7, F7–T3, T3–T5, T5–01; Fp2–F4, F4–C4, C4–P4, P4–02; Fp1–F3, F3–C3, C3–P3 and P3–01

Figure 167 continued

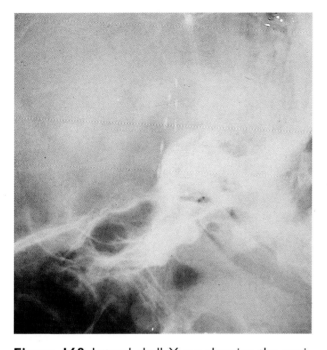

Figure 168 Lateral skull X-ray showing the position of multicontact foramen ovale electrodes. This is a useful means of lateralizing medial temporal seizures, but may provide misleading information if seizures originate elsewhere

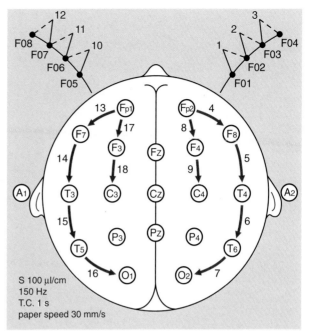

Figure 169 EEGs (below and overleaf) show lateralization of seizures of right medial temporal onset. From top to bottom: F01–F02, F02–F03, F03–F04; Fp2–F8, F8–T4, T4–T6, T6–02; Fp2–F4, F4–C4, F05–F06, F06–F07, F07–F08; Fp1–F7, F7–T3, T3–T5, T5–01; Fp1–F3 and F3–C3

Figure 169 continued

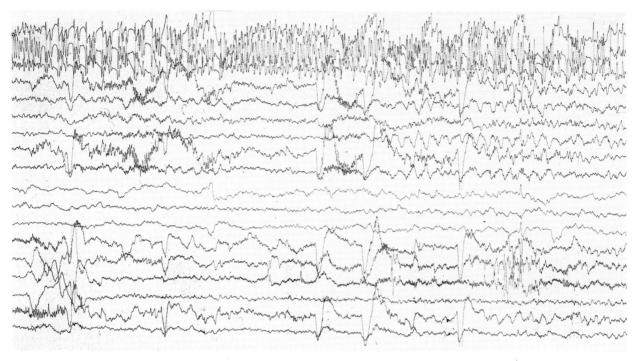

Figure 169 continued From top to bottom: F01–F02, F02–F03, F03–F04; Fp2–F8, F8–T4, T4–T6, T6–02; Fp2–F4, F4–C4, F05–F06, F06–F07, F07–F08; Fp1–F7, F7–T3, T3–T5, T5–01; Fp1–F3 and F3–C3

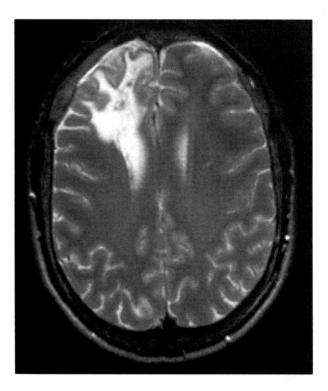

Figure 170 Postinfective scar. At 12 years of age, this boy underwent surgical drainage of a right frontal abscess. He then developed partial and tonic-clonic seizures 2 years later. MRI reveals high-signal material, predominantly in the white matter of the anterior part of the right hemisphere, associated with enlargement of the right frontal horn. The central low-signal area suggests calcification. This is extensive gliosis around an old abscess cavity

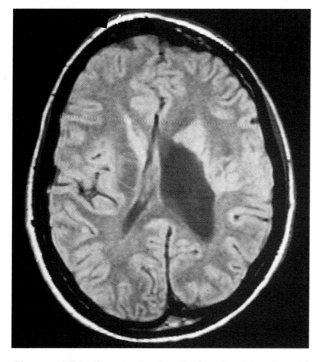

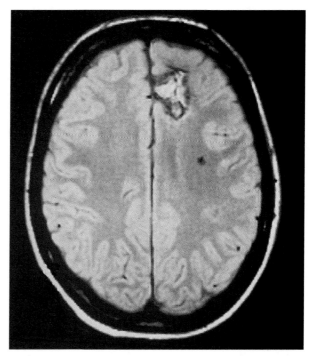

Figure 171 Cortical dysplasia. A 26-year-old woman had drug-resistant complex partial seizures with a right somatosensory aura, and right hemifacial atrophy. MRI shows marked asymmetry of the hemispheres, with enlargement of the left lateral ventricle and a mass of heterotopic gray matter adjacent to the wall of the dilated ventricle. This is the typical appearance of dysplastic brain tissue in association with a neuronal migration disorder

Figure 172 Cavernous angioma. A highly intelligent child developed partial seizures manifested by speech arrest, confusion and bilateral motor automatisms with occasional secondary generalization. Axial MRI with T_2 coronal and proton density demonstrates a partly serpiginous lesion in the left medial frontal region

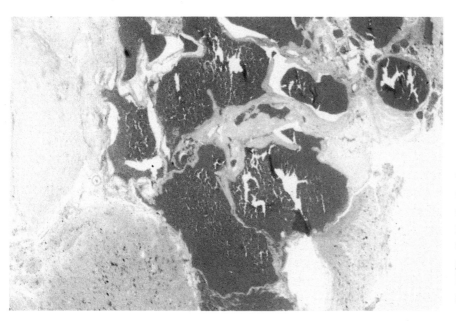

Figure 173 Cavernous hemangioma. Low-power view of the histology shows numerous large dilated venous channels in the leptomeninges on the surface of a temporal lobe, which shows gliosis, focal cavitation and hemosiderin discoloration. (H & E)

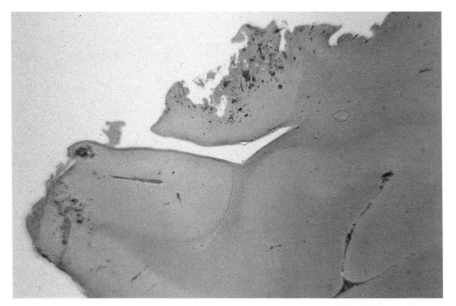

Figure 174 Mesial temporal sclerosis. Histological view of a temporal lobectomy shows the hippocampus to be shrunken and discolored. (H & E–luxol fast blue)

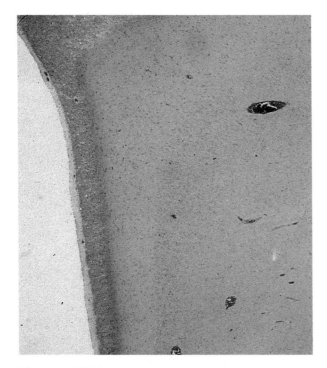

Figure 175 Mesial temporal sclerosis. Higher-power view of the CA1 sector of Figure 174 reveals the complete absence of neurons and the presence of isomorphous gliosis. (H & E–luxol fast blue)

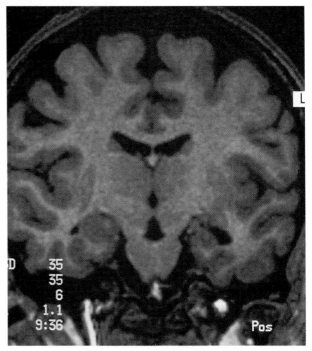

Figure 176 Left hippocampal atrophy. A right-handed woman had experienced prolonged 'febrile' convulsions in association with otitis media at the age of 18 months and refractory complex partial seizures from early childhood. Wada testing revealed right cerebral dominance and impaired left-hemisphere memory function. T$_1$-weighted coronal MRI demonstrates marked hippocampal asymmetry with atrophy of the left side associated with a dilated left temporal horn

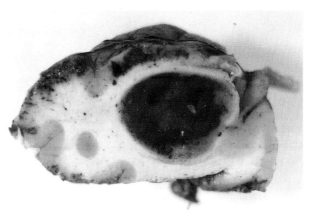

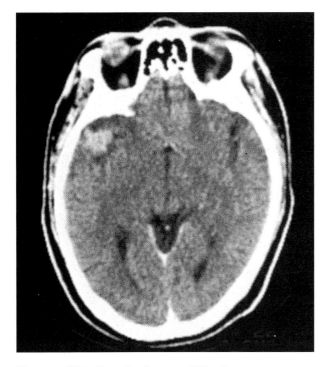

Figure 177 Ganglioglioma. CT of a young man who developed partial seizures at 18 years of age reveals an irregular enhancing lesion in the anterior part of the left temporal lobe. He has remained seizure-free for 3 years following removal of the tumor (see Figure 178)

Figure 178 Ganglioglioma. This resected temporal lobe shows a well-circumscribed tumor; these are the typical appearances and location for a ganglioglioma. Immunocytochemistry of the histology for protein gene product (PGP) 9.5 (lower left) shows several positive-staining well-differentiated neoplastic neurons and processes within a glial background. Immunocytochemistry of the histology for glial fibrillary acidic protein (lower right) reveals the presence of neurons with positive-staining astrocytes. These are an integral constituent of the lesion, but it is not always clear whether or not they are neoplastic

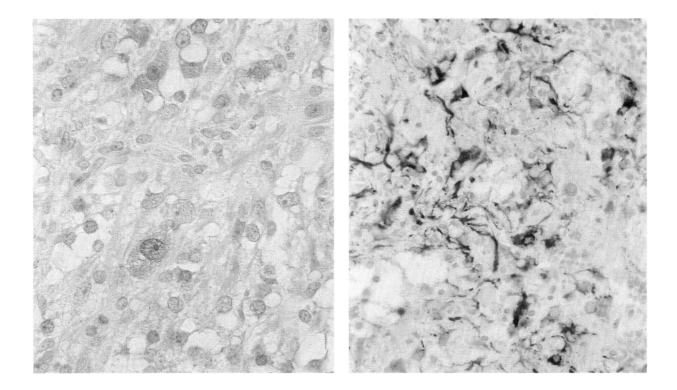

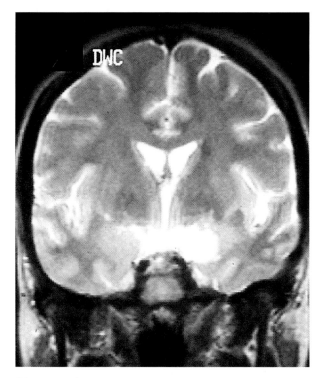

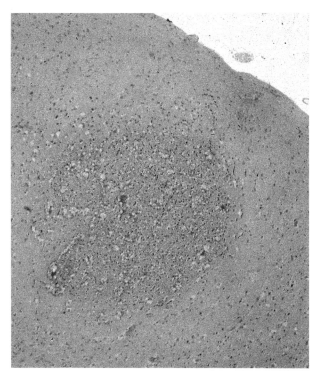

Figure 179 Dysembryoplastic neuroepithelial tumor (DNET). A 23-year-old student presented with a 6-year history of increasingly frequent partial seizures consisting of olfactory hallucinations and expressive dysphasia. T_2-weighted coronal MRI demonstrates a typical high-intensity signal in the left medial temporal lobe

Figure 180 Dysembryoplastic neuroepithelial tumor. Histology of the cerebral cortex shows the characteristically nodular and intracortical architecture of the lesion. (H & E)

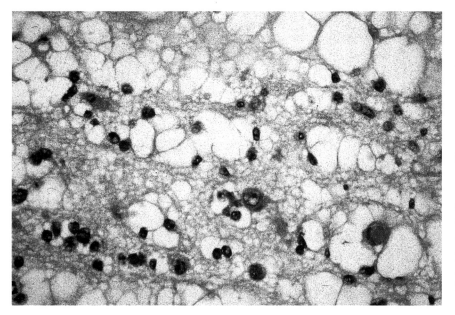

Figure 181 Dysembryoplastic neuroepithelial tumor. High-power view of **Figure 180** shows well-differentiated neurons and glial cells floating in an extracellular matrix. These lesions are biologically indolent and probably hamartomatous. (H & E)

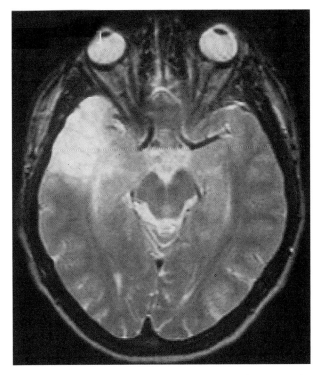

Figure 182 Focal cortical dysplasia. A 23-year-old man had a history of complex partial seizures from the age of 12 years. Wada testing demonstrated defective memory function on the right side. MRI shows an area of hyperintensity involving the anterior and lateral aspects of the right temporal lobe. He remains completely seizure-free 1 year after a right anterior temporal lobectomy

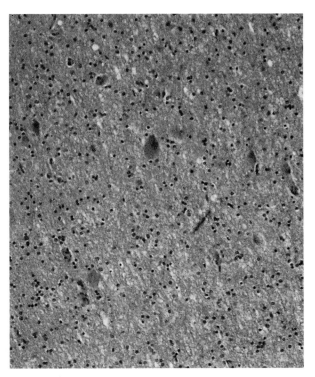

Figure 183 Focal cortical dysplasia. Histology of the cerebral cortex shows disordered architecture with abnormal neurons, some of which are situated in the subcortical white matter. (H & E)

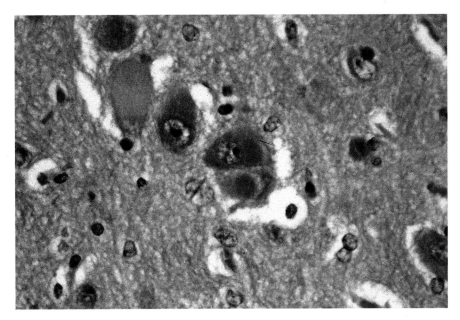

Figure 184 Focal cortical dysplasia. High-power histological view of the cerebral cortex shows morphologically abnormal neurons containing inclusions of cytoskeletal and other subcellular material. (H & E)

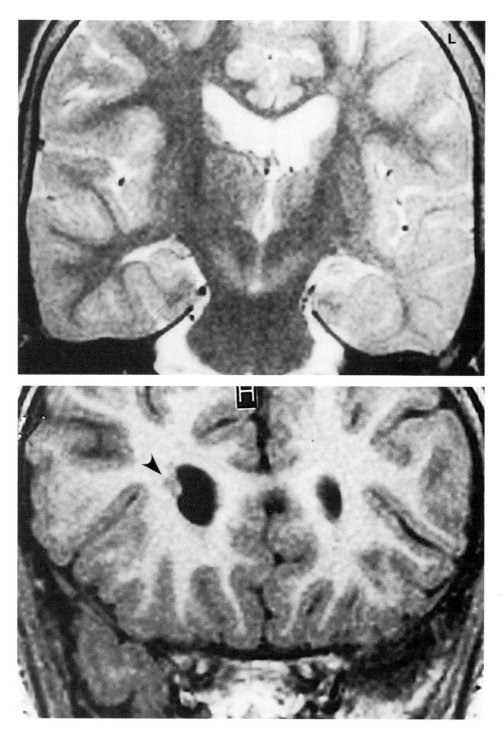

Figure 185 Dual pathology. An 11-year-old girl had a 4-year history of poorly controlled complex partial seizures (with predominantly temporal lobe symptomatology), and no history of 'febrile convulsions' and no cutaneous or radiological stigmata of tuberous sclerosis. T_2-weighted coronal MRI shows hippocampal sclerosis in the left temporal lobe (upper) and subependymal heterotopic gray matter adjacent to, and indenting, the frontal horn of the right lateral ventricle (arrowed; lower). EEG showed only a left temporal slow-wave discharge

Index